STUDY GUIDE

Fifth
EDITION

Foundations *of* Maternal-Newborn and Women's Health Nursing

Sharon Smith Murray, MSN, RN, C

Professor Emerita, Health Professions
Golden West College
Huntington Beach, California

Emily Slone McKinney, MSN, RN, C

Baylor Healthcare System
Dallas, Texas

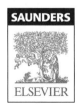

SAUNDERS

ELSEVIER

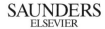

SAUNDERS
ELSEVIER

3251 Riverport Lane
Maryland Heights, Missouri 63043

STUDY GUIDE FOR FOUNDATIONS OF MATERNAL-NEWBORN
AND WOMEN'S HEALTH NURSING, FIFTH EDITION

ISBN: 978-1-4377-0685-7

Notice

Knowledge and best practice in this field are constantly changing. As new research and experience broaden our knowledge, changes in practice, treatment and drug therapy may become necessary or appropriate. Readers are advised to check the most current information provided (i) on procedures featured or (ii) by the manufacturer of each product to be administered, to verify the recommended dose or formula, the method and duration of administration, and contraindications. It is the responsibility of the practitioner, relying on their own experience and knowledge of the patient, to make diagnoses, to determine dosages and the best treatment for each individual patient, and to take all appropriate safety precautions. To the fullest extent of the law, neither the Publisher nor the Authors assume any liability for any injury and/or damage to persons or property arising out of or related to any use of the material contained in this book.

The Publisher

Previous editions copyrighted 2006, 2002, 1998, 1994

Executive Editor: Robin Carter
Senior Developmental Editor: Laurie K. Gower
Publishing Services Manager: Jeff Patterson
Project Manager: Amy Rickles
Cover Designer: Gopalakrishnan Venkatram

Printed in the United States of America

Last digit is the print number: 9 8 7 6 5 4 3 2 1

Preface

The *Study Guide for Foundations of Maternal-Newborn and Women's Health Nursing, 5th edition* has been written to help you grasp the important content in each chapter of the main text. Each chapter in this Study Guide corresponds to the text chapter, having the same number and title. Specific activities vary in each chapter according to its content.

We have included **Learning Activities** that provide a variety of approaches to facilitate learning. The exercises include activities such as matching terms, listing important signs and symptoms, describing medical therapy and nursing measures and their rationales, and labeling illustrations.

Check Yourself questions give you an opportunity to answer multiple-choice items that are similar to those you may encounter on a test at school or on the NCLEX® exam. The questions are a mixture of factual items and higher-level questions that require application of that factual knowledge.

Nursing requires more than textbook knowledge, however. Our **Developing Insight** feature guides you to expand your knowledge as you have your clinical experiences. These activities give you specific directions for comparing and using information that you study in class and in your textbook.

Case Studies give you a chance to "try out" your nursing care with a simulated client. The case studies encourage you to use critical thinking to interpret information given in the situation and select appropriate nursing actions. The case studies can be used by an individual or in a small group. If used in a small group, each member can benefit from the thinking skills of others in the group as they choose and defend their nursing care. In addition, you may often incorporate items such as facility protocols in the simulated client care.

As appropriate to the exercise, we have written the answers at the end of each chapter in the Study Guide. In some cases, we give page references in the text for you to locate the answer.

We wish you well as you pursue your career in nursing. It is a wonderful profession that has brought us much joy. Good luck!

Sharon Smith Murray

Emily Slone McKinney

Contents

Part VI   Women's Health Care

Maternity and Women's Health Care Today

Learning Activities

1. Match each term with its definition (a-h).

_____ Association of Women's Health, Obstetric and Neonatal Nurses (AWHONN)

_____ Capitated care

_____ Clinical pathway

_____ Diagnosis-related group (DRG)

_____ Evidence-based practice

_____ Health maintenance organization (HMO)

_____ Managed care

_____ Preferred provider organization (PPO)

a. Group of health care providers that provide cost-discounted services to a specific group of clients

b. National organization that sets standards for perinatal nurses

c. Federal government plan to pay a fixed amount of money for a specific diagnosis

d. Organization that provides comprehensive health services for a fixed fee

e. Team-oriented plan to define expected client outcomes, length of stay, and expected interventions

f. Payer of health care pays a contracted amount to the providers of care for a specific group of clients

g. Health care plan that uses specific agreements and authorizations to control costs

h. Care based on use of reliable research findings to determine best nursing practice to achieve desired outcomes

2. List five major factors that promoted moving the place of birth from the home to the hospital.

   a.

   b.

   c.

   d.

   e.

3. Describe each of the following settings for childbirth.

   a. Traditional hospital setting

   b. Labor, delivery, and recovery (LDR) rooms

   c. Labor, delivery, recovery, and postpartum (LDRP) rooms

   d. Birth centers

   e. Home births

4. Explain how each of the following factors led to the development of family-centered maternity care.

   a. Consumer demands for involvement in their care

   b. Childbirth education to control labor pain

   c. Research about early parent-newborn contact

5. Describe nursing care that may be encountered in each of these areas of community-based perinatal nursing.
   a. Antepartum high-risk women

   b. Postpartum women

   c. Normal newborns

   d. High-risk newborns

6. Describe the types of problems that each type of nontraditional family may encounter.
   a. Single-parent family

   b. Blended family

   c. Extended family

   d. Same-gender family

   e. Adoptive family

   f. High-risk family

7. Explain how communication characteristics of these cultural groups affect nursing communication.

  a. Southeast Asians
     Voice tone

     Eye contact

     Specially respected groups

     Acceptance of medical therapy

  b. Latinos
     Conversational methods

     Head of household

  c. African-Americans
     Language

  d. Middle Easterners
     Obtaining information

     Interpreters

     Paternalism

  e. Native Americans
     Meaning of a child's behavioral characteristics

     Family characteristics

     Nonmedical influences related to health and illness

8. Draw a graph that shows the most recent differences in white and African-American maternal and infant mortality rates. Use the Internet to obtain the most recent information about these rates.

9. What is the leading cause of death in women in the United States?

10. List three major health problems that are linked to obesity.

Check Yourself

1. If a hospital spends more than expected on a client for care under a specific diagnosis-related group (DRG), the hospital will be
   a. Reimbursed the amount it spent on the client's care
   b. Unable to care for the next client with that condition
   c. Required to absorb the excess costs
   d. Paid more for care of a client with a less costly problem

2. Which of these standards governs the nurse's scope of perinatal nursing practice?
   a. Association of Women's Health, Obstetric and Neonatal Nurses (AWHONN)
   b. Joint Commission on Accreditation of Healthcare Organizations (JCAHO)
   c. The nurse's state nurse practice act
   d. Food and Drug Administration (FDA)

3. A nurse reacts with anger because a woman has not had prenatal care because she does not see pregnancy as an illness that requires health care. The nurse's reaction demonstrates
   a. Cultural diversity
   b. Fatalism
   c. Predestination
   d. Ethnocentrism

4. The major concern about use of complementary or alternative therapies is
   a. Cost that replaces more effective medicines
   b. Safety of some of the treatments used
   c. Questionable advertising by practitioners
   d. Ability to buy herbal preparations over the Internet

Developing Insight

1. Think of a distinctive custom (or behavior, article of clothing, jewelry, etc.) that you have noted in people from a cultural group other than your own. Find out more about the origins of that custom.

2. Discuss health plans with several people. Ask them what, if any, restrictions are placed on their care providers. Determine how much these restrictions concern them and why.

3. What are the proportions of insured and uninsured people in your local area of practice? How do uninsured people obtain essential health care if they seek care? What federal or state laws affect health care?

ANSWERS TO SELECTED QUESTIONS

Learning Activities

1. b, f, e, c, h, d, a, g
2. Births moved from home to hospital because of the (a) discovery that hygienic practices could prevent puerperal infection; (b) development of forceps; (c) discovery of chloroform and drugs to control the pain of childbirth; (d) development of drugs to start or augment labor; (e) development of more operative procedures.
3. (a) Traditional hospital setting: labor, delivery, recovery, and postpartum (LDRP) care occurs in separate rooms; parent-infant contact may be delayed. (b) Labor, delivery, and recovery (LDR) rooms: labor, delivery, and immediate recovery occur in a single room, with transfer to a postpartum room for continuing care; emphasis on keeping parents and infant together; liberal visiting. (c) LDRP rooms: same as LDR rooms, except that mother and infant remain in the same room where birth occurred during the postpartum period. (d) Birth centers: freestanding centers that provide antepartum, intrapartum, postpartum, and newborn care to low-risk mothers and babies; typically staffed by certified nurse-midwives. Basic gynecologic and contraceptive services are often included. (e) Home births: birth occurs in a familiar setting with support people the mother wants; fewer nurse-midwives now attend these births because of malpractice insurance problems.
4. (a) In the 1950s, consumers insisted on their right to be involved in their health care and wanted information and control over birth. (b) Childbirth education gave women options to manage pain while remaining awake and aware. (c) Research showed that benefits of early parent-infant contact outweigh any infection risks.
5. (a) Women with common high-risk conditions, such as preterm labor, hyperemesis gravidarum, bleeding problems, preterm premature rupture of the membranes, hypertension, and diabetes, may receive some home care during pregnancy. (b) Most postpartum home care begins in the birth facility with classes in self-care, closed-circuit television or videos, and provision of written materials in appropriate languages. Individual teaching and return demonstration by the client allow the nurse to determine whether the teaching is adequate or needs supplementation. (c) Phone calls, home visits, information lines, lactation consultants, videotapes, and nurse-managed outpatient clinics. (d) Information and support for technology-dependent infants or infants with congenital anomalies; coordination of care among specialty providers.
6. (a) Poverty, overwhelming responsibilities, less prepared for illness or unemployment. (b) Differences in parenting styles, values, and beliefs about discipline. (c) Generational conflicts. Physical, financial, and emotional stress if grandparents must raise grandchildren because of the inability of the child's parents to do so. (d) Conflict with community values. (e) May have little time to prepare for birth; inadequate support after the adoption. Lack of knowledge about child's health history and developmental or growth delays, need to assimilate a child born in another country, decisions about telling the child about being adopted. (f) Multiple life stressors (see text, including Chapter 24, for greater detail) that may require referral to several community resources and coordination of care.
7. (a) Soft voice; no prolonged eye contact; respect for elderly, priests, and physicians; seldom say no, yet may not follow prescribed treatment if they do not agree. (b) Polite, with preliminary small talk. Male usually the head of household. (c) May use idioms, colloquialisms, or speech patterns that are unfamiliar to health professionals. (d) Information shared only with friends and family; interpreters should be from an acceptable region; paternalism requires male's permission or opinions. (e) Willful children are strong, docile children are weak. Family relationships usually close. Health is state of harmony with nature. Supernatural influences affect health and illness.
8. What kind of graph did you create? Did the activity emphasize the difference between white and African-American infant mortality? What website did you use to obtain the latest information?
9. Cardiovascular disease
10. Hypertension, high blood cholesterol, diabetes mellitus

Check Yourself

1, c; 2, c; 3, d; 4, b

The Nurse's Role in Maternity and Women's Health Care

Learning Activities

1. Describe the education required and services provided by each type of advanced practice nurse is qualified to deliver.
   a. Certified nurse-midwife (CNM)

   b. Nurse practitioners
      (1) Women's health nurse practitioner (WHNP)

      (2) Family nurse practitioner (FNP)

      (3) Neonatal nurse practitioner (NNP)

      (4) Pediatric nurse practitioner (PNP)

   c. Clinical nurse specialist (CNS)

2. A dialog between a woman and a nurse follows. Nonverbal behaviors are in brackets. For each of the nurse's responses, label the communication techniques or blocks that the response illustrates. Explain what feelings you think the client seems to express. If the nurse's response indicates a communication block, write an alternate nursing response.

Situation: A 36-year-old woman is being seen in her gynecologist's office for an annual well-woman checkup.

a. *Nurse:* Well, it's time again for your annual examination, isn't it? Tell me how you have been doing since we last saw you.

   Woman: I haven't had any real problems; I'm doing okay, I suppose . . . [Client looks down at her hands and is silent.]

b. *Nurse:* That's great! We're glad you're doing well, and coming in for a checkup helps keep you that way.

   Woman: I just wish I were coming because I was pregnant.

c. *Nurse:* Are you saying that you want to become pregnant?

   Woman: Well, I'm 36 years old, and time is running out.

d. *Nurse:* Oh, not necessarily. Women have babies even into their 40s. Miracles happen every day.

   Woman: I don't know . . .

e. *Nurse:* You were saying that time is running out. Can you tell me more about your concerns?

   Woman: Well, when I was in my 20s, I wanted to finish graduate school and get established in a career. Then when I was in my early 30s, I just seemed too busy to take time to have a baby. Now... [Her voice trails off.]

f. *Nurse:* [Waiting quietly while the woman gathers her thoughts.] It sounds as if you may regret your decision to wait.

   Woman: Well, my husband and I decided to try to have a baby about 9 months ago. Since I never had trouble with my periods or anything, I thought it would be 3 or 4 months at most until I was pregnant.

g. *Nurse:* Um . . . hmm . . . [Nods and waits quietly.]

Woman: Now I'm afraid my selfishness will keep us from ever having a baby.

h. *Nurse:* Oh, they can do so many things to help couples conceive now. Miracles happen every day.

Woman: That's probably what it will take for me . . . a miracle.

3. Following is a list of the nine principles of teaching and learning. Give an example of how each principle has been used in your own nursing education.
   a. Readiness to learn

   b. Active participation

   c. Skill repetition

   d. Positive feedback

   e. Role modeling

   f. Resolving conflicts and frustration

   g. Simple to complex order

   h. Varied teaching methods

   i. Presenting small segments of information over time

4. List the five steps in critical thinking.

a.

b.

c.

d.

e.

5. Describe differences between a screening assessment and a focused assessment.

a. Screening assessment

b. Focused assessment

6. For each broad goal, write at least three outcome criteria that (1) are client focused, (2) use measurable verbs, (3) have a time frame, and (4) are realistic.

a. After cesarean birth, the woman will have increased mobility.

b. The pregnant woman will have adequate nutrition.

c. The new parents will accept their infant who has a birth defect (cleft lip).

7. For the nursing diagnosis "Ineffective airway clearance related to pain from cesarean birth incision," write four to six specific nursing interventions.

Check Yourself

1. Your friend says she is not sure she wants a physician to deliver her second baby because she believes physicians are too busy to talk with her when she has checkups. The best alternative professional for you to suggest is the
   a. Perinatal nurse practitioner
   b. Certified nurse-midwife
   c. Lay midwife
   d. Clinical nurse specialist

2. A primary difference between social communication and therapeutic communication is that therapeutic communication is
   a. Designed to obtain information in minimal time
   b. The only appropriate professional communication
   c. Focused on achieving a relevant goal for the client
   d. Limited to the information necessary for safe care

3. A pregnant woman tells the nurse, "I'm so confused. My husband wants me to have my tubes tied after the baby comes, but what if something happens to the baby?" The nurse replies, "You're afraid of having permanent contraception before you know if your baby is well." The nurse's response is an example of
   a. Directing
   b. Paraphrasing
   c. Summarizing
   d. Pinpointing

4. The nurse has taught a group of four new mothers how to care for themselves while breastfeeding. At the end of the class, it is most helpful if the nurse
   a. Asks whether the mothers have questions about breastfeeding
   b. Has each mother demonstrate a technique to the other women
   c. Distributes a small gift in return for attending the class
   d. Summarizes the most important points about the lesson

5. A nursing diagnosis differs from a collaborative problem primarily in terms of whether the nurse
   a. Can prescribe definitive treatment for the problem
   b. Identifies a client strength or weakness
   c. Determines that an actual or a potential problem exists
   d. Is able to evaluate the client's response to treatment

Developing Insight

1. In the clinical setting, select a topic that a client or family needs to learn. Use at least three of the principles of teaching and learning in your presentation. Explain how you used each principle in your teaching.

ANSWERS TO SELECTED QUESTIONS

Learning Activities

1. (a) Registered nurses who complete a course of study and clinical experience and are certified by the American College of Nurse-Midwives; they take health histories and perform physical examinations, provide complete care to childbearing families before and after birth, and provide gynecologic services and family planning. (b) Registered nurses with advanced preparation; they provide primary care to clients, including health maintenance and promotion. Nurse practitioners who may be encountered in maternal-newborn and women's health include (1) WHNP: Wellness-focused primary reproductive and gynecologic care; (2) FNP: Preventive and holistic care to young and old, males and females; (3) NNP: Care to high-risk newborns, usually in the neonatal intensive care unit; (4) PNP: Health maintenance of infants and children. (c) Registered nurses with graduate education to be experts in the care of childbearing families; functions include clinical leader, role model, client advocate, and change agent.

2. Techniques (T) or blocks (B) used by the nurse: (a) directing with an open-ended statement (T); (b) failure to acknowledge implied concerns and the client's nonverbal behavior (B); (c) clarifying (T); (d) false reassurance (B); (e) clarifying (T); (f) silence and pinpointing (T); (g) silence (T); (h) false reassurance (B).

3. Reflect on your own education to answer this exercise.

4. (a) Recognition of assumptions that can lead to unexamined thoughts or unsound actions. (b) Examination of personal biases that can sway your mind based on personal theories or stereotypes. (c) Analysis of the amount of pressure for closure that can lead you to a hasty decision based on inadequate information. (d) Examination of data to collect and analyze them more efficiently. (e) Evaluation of the way emotions and environmental factors can interfere with critical thinking (defensiveness, anger, frustration; busy environment).

5. (a) Gathering data about all aspects of a client's health to identify strengths and problems. (b) Gathering additional information focused on an actual problem or one that the client or family is at risk for acquiring.

6. Note: Each outcome criterion is an example of how a nurse might word it; yours may differ and may still be accurate. (a) Sylvia will ambulate in her room by 24 hours after surgery. She will ambulate the length of the hallway and back by 48 hours after surgery. (b) By her next prenatal visit, Jamie will bring a diet journal for 1 day that demonstrates the correct amounts of food from every group on the food pyramid. (c) Gordon and Ginger will hold, make eye contact with, feed, and provide care to their newborn within 24 hours of birth.

7. Your interventions should focus on maintaining adequate pain relief, support of the incision with a pillow when coughing to promote expulsion of secretions, and deep breathing in conjunction with adequate and continuous pain control. The woman needs a combination of both pain control and respiratory management to clear her airway of secretions most effectively. Interventions should also be included to monitor her respiratory status and compare those data with her baseline data. Write four to six specific interventions with these criteria in mind.

Check Yourself

1, b; 2, c; 3, b; 4, d; 5, a

Ethical, Social, and Legal Issues

Learning Activities

1. Match each term with its definition (a-h).

_____ Ethical dilemma

_____ Incident report

_____ Malpractice

_____ Medicaid

_____ Mutual recognition model

_____ Negligence

_____ Statute of limitations

_____ TANF

a. The latest date by which a malpractice suit can be filed

b. Government program that provides money for a limited time for basic living costs of poor children

c. Failure of a professional person to act in a reasonable and prudent way for the circumstances

d. Government program to provide health care to the poor, aged, and disabled

e. A situation in which no solution seems satisfactory

f. Documentation of occurrences that might result in legal action

g. Failure to act as a reasonable, prudent person of similar background would act under similar circumstances

h. Ability of a nurse to be licensed in one state and practice in certain other states based on the same license

2. Describe the differences between the theories that guide ethical decision making.
   a. Deontologic

   b. Utilitarian

3. Define each ethical principle, and give examples of each principle based on your own experience.
   a. Beneficence

   b. Nonmaleficence

   c. Autonomy

   d. Justice

4. Describe provisions of the *Roe v. Wade* U.S. Supreme Court ruling on abortion.
   a. First trimester

   b. Second trimester

   c. Third trimester

5. Working poor is a term that describes people who _____

_____.

6. Why would guaranteed, convenient, and accessible tax-supported prenatal care probably be cheaper for taxpayers?

7. Describe how each of these factors influences nursing practice.
  a. State nurse practice acts

  b. Multistate licensure

  c. Standardized procedures

  d. Standards of care

  e. Agency policies

8. Describe and give an example of each element of negligence.
  a. Duty

  b. Breach of duty

  c. Damage

  d. Proximate cause

9. Describe the four requirements of informed consent.
  a. Competence

  b. Full disclosure

  c. Understanding information

  d. Voluntary

10. How does a long statute of limitations for lawsuits involving a newborn relate to nursing documentation?

Check Yourself

1. A nurse is morally opposed to abortion at any time during pregnancy. Which statement best describes the nurse's responsibility related to this belief?
   a. The nurse must make this position known before being employed at an agency that provides abortions.
   b. The nurse may decline to participate in abortion but must care for women after the procedure.
   c. The nurse cannot accept employment in any agency that may provide abortion services.
   d. The nurse must provide the same care for women undergoing abortion procedures as for any other woman.

2. Poverty tends to be a multigenerational problem because
   a. Poor families often accept their situation as inevitable
   b. Poor children are often discriminated against in school
   c. The women tend to have many closely spaced babies later in life
   d. Dependence on welfare keeps poor women from obtaining an education

3. A nurse who makes a medication error should
   a. Complete an incident report and record this fact in the client's chart
   b. Ask the physician to change the ordered medication to match the one given
   c. Limit care to activities that do not involve giving medications
   d. Chart the medication that was actually given to the client

4. Notations written on a fetal monitor strip
   a. Are a legal part of the chart
   b. Should be kept for 7 years
   c. Replace all client documentation on labor flow sheets
   d. Provide adequate documentation of labor nursing care

Developing Insight

1. In your clinical setting, talk with the staff about ethical dilemmas they have experienced. How were the dilemmas resolved? What policies are in place to help nurses deal with ethical dilemmas?

2. Examine consent forms used in your agency for vaginal and cesarean births, for circumcision, and for anesthesia.

3. What is your agency's chain of command if a physician's response to a nurse's request for instruction is inadequate or inappropriate?

4. What is the typical length of stay in your facility for a woman who delivered vaginally? For a woman who delivered by cesarean birth? For a normal newborn? What steps does your facility take to help mothers and infants cope with early discharge?

5. Look up the latest statistics for the poverty rate on the Internet. How does the rate of poverty differ among different racial groups? Does the incidence of poverty differ when a household is headed by one person rather than two? If the household is headed by one person, do rates differ between those headed by women and those headed by men? Does age make a difference in these statistical numbers? Can you support the reliability of statistics from the Internet site you chose?

ANSWERS TO SELECTED QUESTIONS

Learning Activities

1. e, f, c, d, h, g, a, b

2. (a) Decision is made by using ethical principles and moral rules, without weighing other factors that may have a bearing on the situation. (b) Analyzes the benefits and burdens of a course of action in making an ethical decision; actions may vary according to the situation.

3. (a) Doing or promoting good for others. (b) Avoiding causing harm to others. (c) The right to self-determination, including right to respect, privacy, and information needed to make decisions. (d) Principle that all people should be treated fairly and equally. Draw from your own experiences to give examples. The examples may be from your clinical experiences or from other life experiences.

4. (a) A woman can obtain an abortion at any time. (b) The state can regulate abortions only to protect the woman's health. (c) The state can regulate abortions, except when the mother's life might be jeopardized by continuing the pregnancy.

5. The working poor have jobs, but their wages barely meet daily needs. They may have no insurance coverage in their jobs, or the high cost of coverage may be more than they can pay and meet their day-to-day needs. They often have little or no money in savings.

6. Low-birth-weight infants are more likely to be born to women who did not have prenatal care. Their care and perhaps long-term dependence on technology cost taxpayers millions of dollars.

7. (a) Each state has a nurse practice act that defines what a nurse legally can and cannot do. It is the nurse's responsibility to know his or her state's nurse practice act and practice within those guidelines. (b) States that recognize multistate licensure allow a nurse to practice nursing in the state that issued the license and in states that have agreed to recognize that state's license. (c) Standardized procedures allow nurses with specific education and training to assume duties commonly considered to be part of medical practice. (d) Professional associations describe the standards of care that consumers can expect from practitioners. The specific standards vary according to the practice area. Standards for perinatal and women's health nurses are typically set by AWHONN (Association of Women's Health, Obstetric and Neonatal Nurses). (e) Agency policies set more detailed standards of practice that apply to that specific agency. A nurse who practices in that setting should be familiar with those policies.

8. (a) The nurse must have had a duty to provide care or act on behalf of the client. Example: A nurse should regularly assess the fetal heart and uterine contractions on a fetal monitor strip and take action according to standard practice. (b) The nurse must fail to conform to expected standards of care. Example: The nurse failed to assess the fetal heart and uterine contractions or failed to take appropriate actions. (c) Actual harm came to the client (fetus) because of the nurse's breach of duty. Example: The fetal heart rate decreased to a range of 70 to 80 beats per minute (bpm). Contractions were excessive, and the nurse took no action. (d) The breach of duty (action or inaction) must be proved to be the cause of harm. Example: A jury finds that the child's resulting developmental delay was caused by the nurse's failure to take standard steps to improve fetal oxygenation and reduce excessive contractions.

9. (a) The client must be able to think through a situation and make rational decisions when given the facts. (b) The client must be told what the treatment entails and what the expected results are. Side effects, benefits, and other options must also be disclosed. (c) The information must be presented in a manner that is comprehensible to the client. Interpreters must be used if needed. (d) Only the client can give consent, and this consent must be voluntary rather than forced.

10. The statute of limitations for filing a lawsuit involving a newborn may be many years. The nurse cannot rely on memory of the event but must document in a clear, legible, objective, and complete manner so that the condition of the client and the care given are clear at a much later date.

Check Yourself

1, a; 2, a; 3, d; 4, a

Reproductive Anatomy and Physiology

Learning Activities

1. Match each term with its definition (a-f).

_____ Feedback loop

_____ Linea terminalis

_____ Nocturnal emissions

_____ Perineum

_____ Rugae

_____ Vulva

a. Imaginary line dividing the upper (false) pelvis from the lower (true) pelvis

b. Involuntary release of seminal fluid from the penis during sleep

c. Small ridges or folds of tissue in the female vagina and on the male scrotum

d. Collective term for all the female external reproductive organs

e. Change in the level of one secretion in response to a change in the level of another secretion

f. Posterior part of external female reproductive organs

2. What mechanism prevents onset of puberty before the proper time?

3. The period of maturation of reproductive organs is called _____.

4. a. The first outward change of puberty in girls is _____.
    b. Puberty begins in girls at an average age range of _____ to _____ years.
    c. Girls usually experience their first menstrual period approximately _____ years after the first outward change
    associated with puberty.

5. a. The first outward change of reproductive maturation in boys is _____.
    b. Penile development occurs approximately _____.

6. What factors cause the average male to be taller than the average female at physical maturity?

7. Explain the importance of each type of uterine muscle (myometrial) tissue. Where is each type primarily located?
    a. Longitudinal fibers
        (1) Importance

        (2) Location

    b. Interlacing (figure-eight) fibers
        (1) Importance

        (2) Location

    c. Circular fibers
        (1) Importance

        (2) Location

8. Fertilization normally occurs in the _____.

9. What is the difference in the time when the immature female and male gametes are formed?
   a. Female gametes

   b. Male gametes

10. Match each structure with its functions (a-j). Some letters may be used more than once; other letters may not be used at all. What is the structure that is described by any answer that you do not choose?

_____ Acinar cells

_____ Bartholin's glands

_____ Corpus cavernosum

_____ Corpus spongiosum

_____ Leydig's cells

_____ Montgomery's tubercles

_____ Myoepithelial cells

_____ Perineum

_____ Scrotum

_____ Sertoli cells

_____ Skene's glands

a. Enable erection of the penis for coitus

b. Nourish sperm during their formation within the testes

c. Promote lubrication of the vagina for coitus

d. Produce milk from substances extracted from blood

e. Secrete a substance to keep nipples soft during breastfeeding

f. Regulate temperature of testes to promote normal sperm formation

g. Lubricate the female's urethra

h. Provide support for female pelvic structures

i. Secrete testosterone in the male

j. Discharge milk into the ductal system of the breast

11. Describe events in each phase of the ovarian cycle.
   a. Follicular phase

   b. Ovulatory phase

   c. Luteal phase

12. Describe events in each phase of the menstrual cycle.
   a. Proliferative phase

   b. Secretory phase

   c. Menstrual phase

13. Why might a man who usually wears very tight underwear have a problem with infertility?

LABELING

1. Label each of the external female reproductive structures.

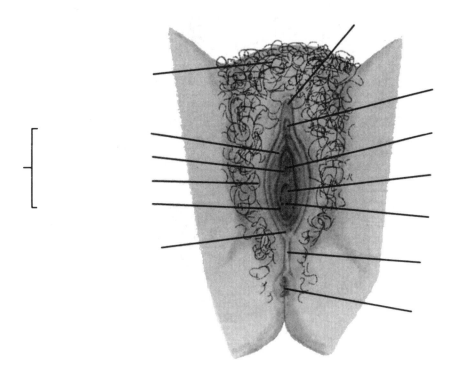

2. Label each of the internal female reproductive structures.

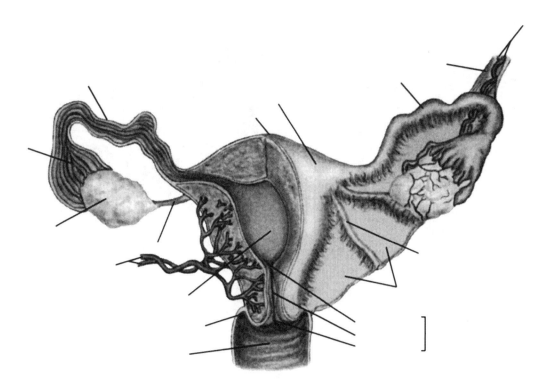

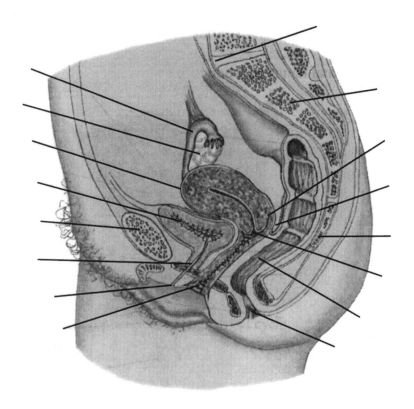

3. Label each landmark on the pelvis.

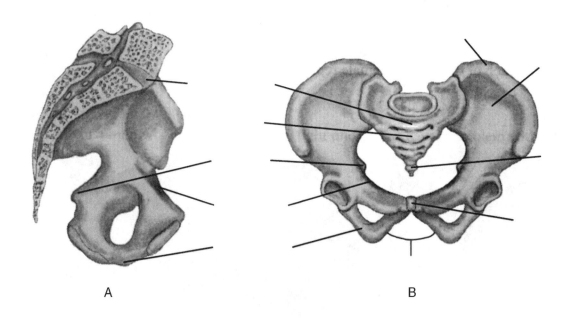

4. Label each muscle and muscle group of the female pelvic floor.

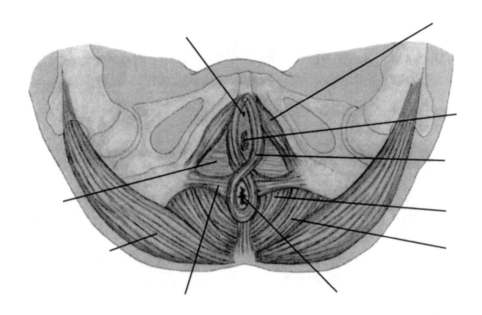

5. Label each structure of the female breast.

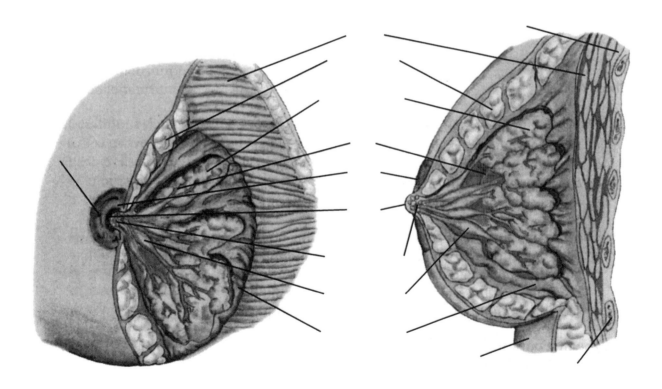

6. Label each structure of the male reproductive system.

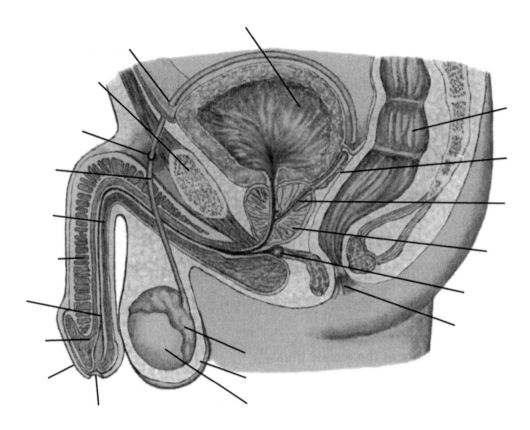

Check Yourself

1. The gender of an infant will be female unless
  a. Two X chromosomes are received from the mother
  b. The short arm of the Y chromosome is received from the father
  c. Conception occurs during the last half of the female reproductive cycle
  d. The mother's ovary produces testosterone early in pregnancy

2. The primary purpose of gonadotropin-releasing hormone (GnRH) is to stimulate
  a. Development of the woman's breasts for lactation
  b. Growth of pubic and axillary hair
  c. Breakdown of the endometrium in the menstrual flow
  d. Secretion of follicle-stimulating hormone (FSH) and luteinizing hormone (LH) from the anterior pituitary gland

3. The first outward change of puberty in girls is
  a. Rapid growth to reach the adult height and weight
  b. Enlargement and development of the breasts
  c. Onset of menstruation
  d. Increase in clear vaginal secretions

4. Choose the girl who is most likely to have secondary amenorrhea.
  a. Amanda, 15 years old, who is trying out for the school track team for girls
  b. Brittney, 17 years old, who is preparing for a national gymnastic tournament
  c. Chloe, 16 years old, who controls type 1 diabetes mellitus with insulin
  d. Deanna, 16 years old, who is a member of an Irish dancing team

5. Males are usually taller than females when they reach their adult height because
   a. Their growth in height occurs early in puberty and continues briefly after puberty
   b. Their secretion of testosterone delays closure of the epiphyses of the long bones
   c. Their puberty changes begin approximately 2 years later than in the average female
   d. The puberty growth spurt begins later and continues for a longer time

6. The layer of uterine muscle that is most active during labor is composed of _____ fibers.
   a. Longitudinal
   b. Interlacing
   c. Circular

7. The layer of uterine tissue that responds to cyclic changes in hormones secreted by the pituitary gland is the
   a. Perimetrium
   b. Myometrium
   c. Endometrium

8. Conditions that cause the fallopian tubes to be narrower than normal may result in
   a. Excessive cramping and bleeding during menstruation
   b. Increased likelihood of pregnancy during each cycle
   c. More rapid propulsion of the ovum through the tube
   d. Implantation of a fertilized ovum within the tube

9. Extra follicles that remain after ovulation
   a. Release their ovum during the last half of the reproductive cycle
   b. Resume maturation during the next reproductive cycle
   c. May be fertilized during another reproductive cycle
   d. Are never active in another reproductive cycle

10. Menstruation occurs because the
   a. Hormone stimulation from the corpus luteum ceases
   b. Blood vessels in the uterine lining become too long and twisted
   c. Corpus luteum increases estrogen and progesterone production
   d. Ovum has been passed from the woman's body

11. Milk is manufactured within the _____ of the breast.
   a. Lactiferous ducts
   b. Alveoli
   c. Myoepithelium
   d. Montgomery's tubercles

12. The primary purpose of the cremaster muscle is to
   a. Eject milk into the lactiferous ducts of the breasts
   b. Maintain the uterus in an anteflexed position
   c. Keep the testes cooler than the rest of the body
   d. Expel seminal fluids to nourish sperm at ejaculation

13. Erection of the penis occurs when
   a. Blood is trapped within the organ's spongy tissue
   b. Warmth allows relaxation of the perineal muscles
   c. Spermatozoa reach 250 million in the testes
   d. The cremaster muscle relaxes on each side

ANSWERS TO SELECTED QUESTIONS

Learning Activities

1. e, a, b, f, c, d
2. An unknown area of the brain prevents the young child's hypothalamus from responding to estrogen and testosterone secretion by the ovaries or testes. Without gonadotropin-releasing hormone from the hypothalamus, further estrogen or testosterone secretion ceases.
3. Puberty
4. (a) Breast development; (b) 8, 13; (c) 2 to 2.5
5. (a) Growth of the testes; (b) 1 year after testicular growth
6. Boys begin their growth acceleration slightly later than girls. Testosterone's effect on closing the epiphyses of the long bones is not as strong as estrogen's effect. Thus boys start their pubertal growth spurt later (when they are taller) and continue growing in height longer than girls.
7. (a) Longitudinal fibers: importance—expel the fetus at birth; location—fundus. (b) Interlacing fibers: importance—compress blood vessels to prevent hemorrhage after birth; location—middle layer. (c) Circular fibers: importance—prevent reflux of menstrual blood from the uterus into the fallopian tubes, control entry of the embryo into the uterus for implantation, and retain the fetus until proper time for birth; location—constriction around fallopian tubes and internal cervical os.
8. Fallopian tubes
9. (a) Female ova are produced only during prenatal life. (b) Male spermatozoa are produced continuously after puberty.
10. d, c, a, a, i, e, j, h, f, b, g

11. (a) Estrogen and progesterone levels fall just before menstruation, causing increasing secretion of follicle-stimulating hormone (FSH) and luteinizing hormone (LH) by the anterior pituitary; follicles mature with increasing estrogen secretion until one follicle outgrows all others. (b) Marked increase in LH secretion, a slight fall in follicular estrogen, and a rise in follicular progesterone secretion; final maturation and release of the most mature ovum. (c) The corpus luteum secretes progesterone to prepare the endometrium for a fertilized ovum; corpus luteum will persist and continue to secrete progesterone if it receives a signal (human chorionic gonadotropin) from a fertilized ovum. Otherwise, progesterone secretion falls and menstruation occurs.
12. (a) Cells of the basal layer of the endometrium multiply; endometrial glands form; spiral arteries and endometrial veins elongate. (b) Endometrium continues to thicken; substances are secreted to nourish an embryo if one implants. (c) Vasospasm occurs if the corpus luteum stops producing estrogen and progesterone, causing the endometrium to become necrotic. The necrotic layer separates from the basal layer to produce menstrual flow.
13. Tight underwear keeps the testes very near the body, possibly overheating them and suppressing normal sperm development.

Labeling

Refer to these figures in the text to complete this exercise: 1, 4-1; 2, 4-2 and 4-3; 3, 4-5; 4, 4-6; 5, 4-8; 6, 4-9.

Check Yourself

1, b; 2, d; 3, b; 4, b; 5, d; 6, a; 7, c; 8, d; 9, d; 10, a; 11, b; 12, c; 13, a

Hereditary and Environmental Influences on Childbearing

Learning Activities

1. Match each term with its definition (a-j).

_____ Allele

a. Normal gene variation

_____ Karyotype

b. Cells that have added sets of chromosomes

_____ Monosomy

c. Alternate gene form

_____ Mutation

d. Variation in a gene that affects its function

_____ Polymorphism

e. Chromosomes arranged from largest to smallest pairs

_____ Polyploidy

f. One extra chromosome present in each body cell

_____ Somatic cell

g. All or part of a chromosome attached to another

_____ Teratogen

h. Nonreproductive body cell

_____ Translocation

i. Cells that have one missing chromosome

_____ Trisomy

j. Agent that causes or increases the risk for a birth defect

2. Explain how DNA, genes, and chromosomes are related.

3. List the ways genes can be studied.
   a.

   b.

   c.

4. What tissues are used to study genes?
   a.

   b.

   c.

   d.

5. What are some potential implications of the Human Genome Project (HGP)?

6. List the cells that can be used to study chromosomes.
   a.

   b.

   c.

   d.

7. How should the nurse care for specimens used to analyze chromosomes during metaphase?

Why is this care needed?

How does fluorescent in-situ hybridization differ in chromosome analysis?

8. For each type of single gene abnormality, describe the conditions necessary for a child to be affected and specify any gender differences.
   a. Autosomal dominant

   b. Autosomal recessive

   c. X-linked recessive

9. Describe each type of chromosome abnormality.
   a. Numeric

   b. Structural

10. Describe two characteristics that are typical of multifactorial birth defects.
   a.

   b.

11. What factors influence the risk for occurrence of a multifactorial disorder?
  a.

  b.

  c.

  d.

  e.

12. Describe what the nurse should teach a pregnant woman about each classification of possible teratogens.
  a. Infections

  b. Drugs, both therapeutic and illicit

  c. Radiologic procedures

  d. Hot tubs, saunas

13. Describe nursing care related to genetics and birth defects for each of these settings.
  a. Women's health

  b. Antepartum

  c. Intrapartum/neonatal

  d. Pediatrics

Check Yourself

1. The nurse notes 46, XY on the chromosome study of an infant with a birth defect. This means that the infant has
   a. Abnormal genes in all 46 chromosomes
   b. A normal male chromosome analysis
   c. An abnormal female chromosome makeup
   d. Down syndrome (trisomy 21)

2. The nurse should expect a pregnant African-American woman to be offered genetic testing for which disorder?
   a. Cystic fibrosis
   b. Tay-Sachs disease
   c. Rh isoimmunization
   d. Sickle cell trait

3. Loretta and Louis have a child with an autosomal recessive disorder. They want to know whether the problem is likely to recur if they have another child. The nurse should understand that
   a. It is unlikely that they would ever have another child with that abnormality
   b. Each pregnancy has a 1 in 4 (25%) chance of resulting in another affected child
   c. Any pregnancy that occurs before Loretta is 40 years old is unlikely to have the defect
   d. Their risks for having another child with the defect cannot be calculated exactly

4. A woman who is 5 weeks pregnant asks the nurse whether she can take a specific medication to relieve her cold symptoms. The nurse's answer should be based primarily on
   a. Whether the drug is prescription or over-the-counter
   b. The severity of the woman's respiratory symptoms
   c. The pregnancy category of the drug
   d. How long the woman has had the cold

5. A woman who has phenylketonuria (PKU) is considering becoming pregnant. The nurse should teach her that she should expect to
   a. Follow her low-phenylalanine diet before conception and throughout pregnancy
   b. Limit her consumption of foods that are high in phosphates during the first 3 months
   c. Avoid becoming pregnant because her disorder will intensify during pregnancy
   d. Increase her consumption of fluids to speed excretion of phenylalanine

Developing Insight

1. List the blood type and Rh factor of several people you know. Determine the possible combinations of genes that could have produced each.

2. Draw a three-generation pedigree of your family tree, using the symbols on p. 75. Note any traits (normal or abnormal) that you know about in each person. Do you see any patterns?

3. In the clinical setting, review charts for women, infants, children, or families who were referred for some type of genetic studies or counseling. What was the reason? What was the outcome of the counseling?

4. Locate current information about the Human Genome Project (HGP) from the Internet. One resource is the official site: www.genome.gov. Plan a group or individual project on the HGP to present to your clinical group or class. Identify the latest findings on a topic, possible ethical issues, and the future direction of study.

ANSWERS TO SELECTED QUESTIONS

Learning Activities

1. c, e, i, d, a, b, h, j, g, f
2. *DNA* is the basic building block of genes. It resembles a ladder, with a sugar and phosphate group forming the sides of the ladder and pairs of nitrogen bases forming the rungs. Specific segments of DNA form a *gene*, and many genes form a *chromosome.*
3. (In any order) (a) Measuring the products they direct the cells to produce. (b) Direct study of the DNA. (c) Analyzing the gene's linkage with another gene that can be studied in one of the other two ways.
4. (a) Blood; (b) skin cells; (c) hair follicles; (d) fetal cells
5. (a) Direct testing for a disorder or carrier status, which is more accurate than some available tests. (b) Molecular testing for a gene for anyone, not just a person with a family history. (c) Improved accuracy of preconception or prenatal testing for reproductive decisions. (d) Availability of testing to identify one's predisposition to a disorder, thus allowing lifestyle or other changes to reduce risk. (e) Gene therapy. (f) Modifying therapy based on the person's genetic code. (g) Individualizing treatment or medication protocols.
6. (a) White blood cells; (b) skin fibroblasts; (c) bone marrow cells; (d) fetal cells from the chorionic villi or from amniotic fluid
7. Cells must be living and dividing for chromosome analysis during metaphase of cell division. Temperature extremes, blood clotting, or use of improper preservatives can kill the cells. Fluorescent in-situ hybridization does not require active cell division.
8. (a) The child must receive a copy of the autosomal dominant gene from a parent who either is affected or has had a mutation in the germ cell; no gender difference. (b) The child must receive a copy of the autosomal recessive gene from each parent; no gender difference. (c) The child must receive the abnormal gene from the mother. Females are carriers; males are affected because they do not have a compensating normal X chromosome as females do.
9. (a) Numeric: a single chromosome missing or added in every cell or multiple sets of chromosomes. (b) Structural: part of the chromosome is missing or duplicated, or the DNA is rearranged.
10. (a) Those that are present and detectable at birth; (b) single isolated defects
11. Any sequence is acceptable: (a) number of affected close relatives; (b) severity of disorder in affected family members; (c) gender of affected persons; (d) geographic location; (e) season
12. (a) Be immunized or avoid situations in which the potential for acquiring infection is increased. (b) Eliminate use of nontherapeutic or nonessential drugs and other substances; use alternative therapeutic drugs, if possible; use lowest possible dose. (c) Perform during the first 2 weeks after a menstrual period, delay nonurgent procedures until after birth, and shield the abdomen as much as possible if unable to delay the procedure. (d) Avoid or limit exposure, especially at public facilities.
13. (a) Identifying those who can benefit from genetic counseling based on histories and physicals. (b) Identifying those who might benefit from counseling and providing support for their decision making; teaching; helping them deal with abnormal results. (c) Evaluating the family's perception of any problem; helping them understand diagnostic tests; reinforcing correct information; correcting misunderstandings; listening; making referrals to lay support groups. (d) Reducing stress by making referrals to appropriate support services and lay support groups.

Check Yourself

1, b; 2, d; 3, b; 4, c; 5, a

Learning Activities

1. Match each term with its definition (a-j).

_____ Autosome

_____ Blastocyst

_____ Corpus luteum

_____ Decidua

_____ Gamete

_____ Hydramnios

_____ Morula

_____ Oligohydramnios

_____ Polar body

_____ Somatic cell

a. Preembryonic structure that has an outer cell layer and an inner cell mass

b. Uterine endometrium during pregnancy

c. Nonsex chromosome

d. Reproductive cell

e. Ordinary body cell

f. Nonfunctional form to carry away extra chromosomes during oogenesis

g. Cells that remain after ovum formation and secrete estrogen and progesterone

h. Solid ball of 12 to 16 cells formed after fertilization

i. Abnormally large quantity of amniotic fluid

j. Abnormally small quantity of amniotic fluid

2. Compare mitosis to meiosis in the following ways.

	Mitosis	*Meiosis*
a. Type of cell involved		
b. Number and type of chromosomes in each resulting cell		

3. What is *crossing over,* and what is its significance?

4. Compare oogenesis with spermatogenesis in the following ways.

Factor	*Oogenesis*	*Spermatogenesis*
Number and type of chromosomes in each mature gamete		
Number of gametes resulting from each primary cell		
When during life gametogenesis begins and ends		

5. What are the major occurrences immediately after fertilization?
  a.

  b.

  c.

6. List three reasons why the fundus is the best area for implantation.

a.

b.

c.

7. List the three germ layers and the structures that develop from each.

a.

b.

c.

8. State when during prenatal development each event occurs.

a. Closure of the neural tube

b. Heart contains four chambers

c. All abdominal organs are within the abdominal cavity

d. Eyes close: _____ weeks; reopen: _____ weeks

e. External ear development begins

f. Fetal gender apparent by external genitalia

g. Fetal movements felt by mother

h. Surfactant production begins

i. Testes begin entry into scrotum

9. Describe each of these fetal structures or substances, and state its purpose.
   a. Vernix caseosa

   b. Lanugo

   c. Brown fat

   d. Surfactant

10. What is the difference between the fertilization age and the gestational age?

11. Explain how each of the following mechanisms allows the fetus to thrive in the relatively low-oxygen environment of the uterus.
   a. Fetal hemoglobin and hematocrit

   b. Relative fetal and maternal blood carbon dioxide levels

12. Describe how passage of maternal immunoglobulin G (IgG) antibodies can be either beneficial or harmful to the fetus.
   a. Beneficial

   b. Harmful

13. Explain the function of each placental hormone.
   a. Human chorionic gonadotropin (hCG)

   b. Human placental lactogen (hPL)

   c. Estrogen

   d. Progesterone

14. State the three functions of amniotic fluid.

    a.

    b.

    c.

15. Explain the umbilical cord structures and their functions.

    a. Umbilical vein

    b. Umbilical arteries (two)

    c. Wharton's jelly

16. On the following drawing, label each fetal structure. Trace the circulatory route from oxygenated blood in the placenta through the fetal circulation and the return of deoxygenated blood to the placenta.

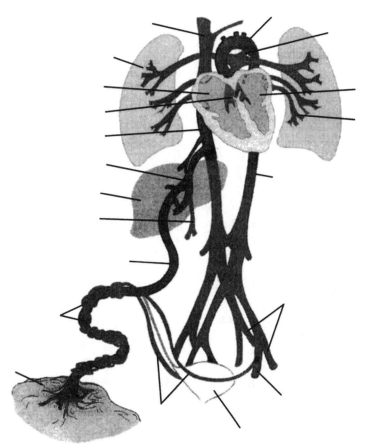

Fetal circulation

17. Explain factors that cause each of these fetal circulatory shunts to close after birth and the eventual outcome for each.
   a. Foramen ovale

   b. Ductus arteriosus

   c. Ductus venosus

18. Describe monozygotic and dizygotic twinning in the following terms.

	Monozygotic	*Dizygotic*
a. Number of ova and sperm involved		
b. Genetic component		
c. Gender		
d. Hereditary tendency		
e. Number of amnions and chorions		

Check Yourself

1. An important purpose of seminal fluid is to
   a. Digest microorganisms in the female reproductive tract
   b. Prevent premature movement of sperm tails
   c. Protect sperm from the acidic vaginal environment
   d. Transport the sperm into the uterine cavity

2. Fertilization is complete when
   a. Fusion of the sperm and ovum nuclei occurs
   b. A sperm enters the ovum in the fallopian tube
   c. The fertilized ovum has its first cell division
   d. The morula fully implants into the uterine lining

3. The embryo is fully implanted in the uterus on which day after conception?
   a. 3
   b. 6
   c. 10
   d. 15

4. Which fetal circulatory structure carries blood with the highest oxygen concentration?
   a. Umbilical artery
   b. Umbilical vein
   c. Ductus arteriosus
   d. Pulmonary vein

5. What substance is the primary energy source for the fetus?
   a. Glucose
   b. Urea
   c. Protein
   d. Fatty acids

6. What is the significance of a fetal hemoglobin of 13 g and a hematocrit of 39%?
   a. Fetal blood is more likely to clot as it circulates through the placenta.
   b. Greater transfer of carbohydrates will result in rapid fetal growth.
   c. Transfer of harmful substances from the mother to the fetus is lessened.
   d. Anemia reduces the oxygen-carrying capacity of the fetal blood.

Developing Insight

1. A woman thinks she is pregnant but begins "spotting" (light vaginal bleeding). Her hCG levels are very low. What is the likely consequence of the low hCG level? Why?

2. Talk to a nurse or neonatal nurse practitioner in the neonatal intensive care unit about the use of artificial surfactant for preterm infants. Which infants are most likely to receive this therapy? Are other measures used to accelerate fetal lung development if preterm birth is likely?

ANSWERS TO SELECTED QUESTIONS

Learning Activities

1. c, a, g, b, d, i, h, j, f, e
2. Mitosis: (a) somatic cell; (b) 46 chromosomes (44 autosomes and two sex [X and Y or two X] chromosomes). Meiosis: (a) gamete (reproductive cell); (b) 23 chromosomes (22 autosomes and either an X [in either a sperm or an ovum] or a Y [only in a sperm].
3. Crossing over allows genetic variation while keeping the total number of chromosomes correct.
4. See Table 6-1 to complete this exercise.
5. (a) The zona pellucida prevents other sperm from entering. (b) The cell membranes of the ovum and sperm fuse and break down. (c) The ovum completes its second meiotic division.
6. (In any order) (a) Good blood supply, (b) thick uterine lining, (c) interlacing muscle fibers to limit postbirth blood loss
7. See Table 6-3 on p. 98 to complete this exercise.
8. See Table 6-2 and the text on pp. 95-100 to answer this question. (a) 4 weeks; (b) 6 weeks; (c) 10 weeks; (d) close: 10 weeks; reopen: 26 to 28 weeks; (e) 6 weeks; (f) 12 weeks; (g) 16 to 24 weeks; (h) 20 weeks; (i) 26 weeks
9. (a) Creamy skin covering to lubricate and protect fetal skin from amniotic fluid. (b) Fine, downy hair that helps vernix adhere to the skin. (c) Heat-producing fat found in back of the neck, behind sternum, and around kidneys. (d) Surface-active lipid substance that helps alveoli remain slightly open between breaths to ease the work of air breathing.
10. Fertilization age is calculated in weeks from the actual time of conception. Gestational age is calculated from the first day of the woman's last menstrual period. Gestational age is approximately 2 weeks longer than fertilization age.
11. (a) High fetal hemoglobin and hematocrit give the fetus more oxygen-carrying capacity; fetal hemoglobin also can carry 20% to 50% more oxygen than adult hemoglobin. (b) Fetal carbon dioxide quickly diffuses into the mother's blood, causing her blood to become more acidic and fetal blood to become more alkaline; this allows fetal blood to combine with oxygen more readily.
12. (a) Provides the newborn with temporary passive immunity to diseases to which the mother is immune. (b) Maternal blood-type antibodies may cross the placenta and destroy incompatible fetal erythrocytes.

13. (a) Causes persistence of the corpus luteum to maintain estrogen and progesterone secretion during early pregnancy and causes fetal testes to secrete testosterone to stimulate development of normal male reproductive structures. (b) Promotes normal growth and nutrition of the fetus, stimulates maternal breast development, and makes more glucose available to fetus by reducing maternal insulin sensitivity and glucose utilization. (c) Causes uterine and breast enlargement, growth of the ductal system of the breasts, and enlargement of fetal external genitalia. (d) Changes endometrium into decidua to nourish conceptus before placenta is established; reduces uterine contractions; may cause the mother's immune system to better tolerate the fetus; acts with estrogens and other hormones to cause growth of the breasts, budding of the alveoli that secrete milk, and development of the secretory characteristics in the alveolar cells of the breasts.
14. (a) Cushions fetus from impacts. (b) Provides stable temperature. (c) Promotes normal fetal growth and development (promotes symmetric development, preventing membrane adherence, and allows fetal movement).
15. (a) Carries oxygenated blood and nutrients from the placenta to the fetus. (b) Carry deoxygenated blood and waste products from the fetus to the placenta. (c) Protects the cord vessels from stretching or pressure that would interrupt flow.
16. See Figure 6-9, *A*, p. 106 to complete this exercise.
17. (a) As infant breathes, resistance to blood flow to lungs falls and the foramen ovale closes; tissue proliferation causes it to fill in the septum between the right and left atria. (b) Rising arterial oxygen levels cause constriction; becomes a ligament. (c) Cessation of umbilical cord blood flow with birth causes it to become nonfunctional; becomes a ligament.
18. (a) Monozygotic: one ovum and one sperm; dizygotic: two ova and two sperm. (b) Monozygotic: identical genes; dizygotic: like any other siblings. (c) Monozygotic: same gender; dizygotic: may be same or different genders. (d) Monozygotic: no hereditary influence known; dizygotic: maternal age and hereditary and ethnic tendencies often found. (e) Monozygotic: numbers of amnions and chorions vary according to the time when the inner cell mass divides in two, but most often two amnions and one chorion; dizygotic: always has two amnions and two chorions.

Check Yourself

1, c; 2, a; 3, c; 4, b; 5, a; 6, d

Physiologic Adaptations to Pregnancy

Learning Activities

1. Match each term with its definition (a-h).

_____ Ballottement

_____ Hyperemia

_____ Lightening

_____ Melasma

_____ Physiologic anemia of pregnancy

_____ Primipara

_____ Quickening

_____ Striae gravidarum

a. Descent of the fetus into the pelvis, reducing pressure on the diaphragm

b. Excess blood in a body part

c. Woman who has given birth once after a pregnancy of at least 20 weeks

d. Irregular reddish streaks caused by tears in connective tissue— stretch marks

e. Fall in hemoglobin and hematocrit that occurs because plasma volume expands more than red blood cell volume

f. First fetal movements felt by the mother

g. Brownish discoloration of the face

h. Fetal rebound in the amniotic fluid when the cervix is tapped

2. On the following figure, label the line that indicates the fundal height at each time during pregnancy.

_____ 8 weeks

_____ 16 weeks

_____ 20 weeks

_____ 26 weeks

_____ 32 weeks

_____ 36 weeks

_____ After lightening has occurred

3. When during pregnancy does each of these markers in fundal height occur?
   a. Uterus can first be palpated above the symphysis pubis

   b. Fundus can be palpated about halfway between the symphysis pubis and umbilicus

   c. Fundus is at level of umbilicus

   d. Fundus is at xiphoid process

4. Describe and give the cause of each of the following changes in the cervix during pregnancy.
   a. Chadwick's sign

   b. Goodell's sign

   c. Hegar's sign

   d. Mucus plug

   e. Bloody show

5. What is the possible result of each of the following changes in the vagina during pregnancy?
   a. Increase in vascularity

   b. Softening of connective tissue

   c. Secretion of increased amounts of glycogen

6. a. Why is progesterone essential in pregnancy?

   b. Progesterone is produced first by the _____ and then by the _____.

7. What pregnancy-induced changes in pigmentation may occur in the following areas? What hormones are responsible?
   a. Face

   b. Breasts

   c. Abdomen

8. What breast changes occur during pregnancy?

9. Describe changes in maternal heart sounds that may occur during pregnancy.
   a. When do the heart sound changes occur?

   b. Describe common changes in heart sounds.

10. What is supine hypotensive syndrome, and what signs and symptoms might a woman with this syndrome display? What should the nurse do to prevent or relieve it?

11. Complete the following chart to describe changes in the pregnant woman's blood.

Component	Change during Pregnancy	Effect
Plasma volume		
Red blood cell mass		
Leukocyte count		
Clotting factors		

12. Why does the pregnancy-induced change in fibrinogen levels and other clotting factors have a protective effect yet also increases risk?

13. What changes allow the woman to obtain the increased oxygen needed during pregnancy?

14. What factors contribute to a woman's sense of dyspnea?

15. What nasal changes are common during pregnancy? What causes them?

16. What causes the heartburn that often occurs in pregnancy?

17. Why are pregnant women more likely to develop gallstones?

18. What changes in the urinary system make the pregnant woman more susceptible to infection?

19. Why does the pregnant woman's bone mass stay stable even though the fetus requires calcium for skeletal development?

20. What changes in carbohydrate metabolism and the production of, utilization of, and sensitivity to insulin occur during pregnancy? Why do these changes occur? How does the woman's body normally respond to these changes?

21. List the presumptive, probable, and positive indications of pregnancy. What are the differences among the three classifications?

Presumptive	Probable	Positive

22. Define the sounds heard when the uterus is auscultated during pregnancy, and specify the heart rate to which each sound corresponds.
    a. Uterine souffle

    b. Funic souffle

23. At what point in gestation is it possible to hear fetal heart sounds with the following tools?
    a. Doppler

    b. Fetoscope

24. What is the difference between gravida and para?

25. Use Nägele's rule to calculate estimated dates of delivery (EDDs) for each of these dates, which represent the first day of the last normal menstrual periods.
 a. February 4

 b. August 2

26. Why is pregnancy risk assessment not a one-time evaluation?

27. What routine urine testing is done during prenatal visits?

28. How does each of the following differ when a woman has a multifetal pregnancy?
 a. Uterine size

 b. Fetal movements

 c. Weight gain

29. Describe significant maternal changes that occur in a multifetal pregnancy.
   a. Blood volume

   b. Cardiac workload

   c. Respiratory effect

   d. Blood vessel compression

   e. Ureter compression

   f. Bowel

30. What teaching is appropriate for each of these common discomforts of pregnancy?
   a. Nausea and vomiting

   b. Heartburn

   c. Backache

   d. Round ligament pain

   e. Urinary frequency

   f. Varicosities

   g. Hemorrhoids

   h. Constipation

   i. Leg cramps

31. What should the pregnant woman be taught about the following practices during pregnancy? How would you explain this to a woman if you were the nurse?

    a. Hot tubs and saunas

    b. Douching

    c. Exercise

    d. Sexual activity

    e. Use of a seat belt

    f. Working

    g. Over-the-counter drugs

    h. Tobacco

    i. Alcohol

    j. Illegal drugs

Check Yourself

1. A pregnant woman expects to give birth to her first baby in approximately 1 week. She asks the nurse whether she has a bladder infection, because she urinates so much, even though urination causes no discomfort. The nurse should explain to her that
    a. Her urine will be tested because urinary tract infections are common in pregnancy
    b. Her fetus is probably lower in her pelvis, and this puts more pressure on her bladder
    c. She should limit her fluid to reduce the number of times she must urinate
    d. Frequent urination is a sign that labor will probably start in a few days

2. The nurse will be concerned about anemia that is not physiologic anemia of pregnancy if a woman in her second trimester has a hemoglobin level less than
  a. 10.5 g
  b. 11 g
  c. 12 g
  d. 13 g

3. Slight hyperventilation during pregnancy enhances
  a. Growth of fetal arteries within the placenta
  b. The fall in systolic and diastolic blood pressures
  c. Maternal metabolism of food and nutrients
  d. Transfer of fetal carbon dioxide to maternal blood

4. A pregnant woman is prone to urinary tract infection primarily because
  a. A large volume of fetal wastes must be excreted by her kidneys
  b. Nutrients that enhance bacterial growth are excreted by her kidneys
  c. The woman voids in frequent small amounts throughout the day and night
  d. Reduced blood flow to the urinary tract allows wastes to accumulate

5. A pregnant woman complains that her hands become numb at times. Neither hand is inflamed or discolored. The nurse should explain to the woman that
  a. She probably injured her hands and does not recall doing so
  b. Undiagnosed fractures may have healed improperly
  c. Osteoarthritis often has its onset during pregnancy
  d. Increased tissue fluid is causing compression of a nerve

6. A pregnant woman has a blood glucose screening at 26 weeks of gestation. The result is 128 mg/dl. The nurse should expect that
  a. No additional glucose testing will be needed
  b. Insulin injections will be needed by 30 weeks of gestation
  c. Oral drugs may be prescribed to lower her glucose level
  d. More testing is needed to determine appropriate therapy

7. Mrs. J. tells you she occasionally has a sharp pain in her right side. The pain does not last long but worries her. You should tell her that
  a. She is probably having appendicitis attacks and may need surgery right away
  b. She may have exercised too much and should take it easy for a few days
  c. She should bend toward the pain or sharply flex her leg to relax the round ligament
  d. Daily twisting and bending exercises will prevent the recurrence of the pain

8. A pregnant woman asks the nurse about skin changes during her pregnancy. The nurse tells her that
  a. The striae will fade to silvery lines
  b. Sunshine will help lighten the melasma
  c. The linea nigra will darken over time
  d. Women with dark skin tones have less hyperpigmentation

Developing Insight

1. Enlist a pregnant woman, and assess her blood pressure in each of the following ways. Allow at least 2 minutes between readings. Compare the systolic and diastolic pressures.
  a. Lateral recumbent position
  b. Sitting with arm supported
  c. Sitting with arm dependent
  d. Standing

    e. Diastolic pressure at sound muffling (Korotkoff's fourth phase)

    f. Diastolic pressure at disappearance of sounds (Korotkoff's fifth phase)

2. Compare a prenatal clinic's documentation forms for initial and subsequent antepartum visits with the recommended assessments listed in the text. What is that clinic's usual recommended frequency for follow-up prenatal visits? Is it different for primigravidas and multigravidas?

3. Talk with nurses at a local prenatal clinic to determine different cultural groups that they typically serve. Ask them how they incorporate cultural beliefs and values into care.

4. Interview a woman who is newly pregnant or planning to become pregnant soon and determine what risk factors she may have. Develop a plan for reducing risk factors where that is possible.

Case Study

Katherine, 36 years old, is making her first antepartum visit on August 12. She has a 2-year-old son who was delivered at 40 weeks, a 7-year-old daughter delivered at 35 weeks, and a 5-year-old daughter delivered at 38 weeks. She states that she had a miscarriage 3 years ago when she was 2½ months pregnant. Her last menstrual period was April 5. Her fundal height is 20 cm. She denies any major complaints and says her health has been good. Katherine is very thin and states she weighed 44 kg (97 lb) before her pregnancy began. She is 160 cm (63 in) tall. She admits to smoking one-half pack per day but denies using drugs or alcohol.

1. Determine Katherine's gravida and para. Describe her obstetric history with the GTPAL acronym.

2. What is Katherine's EDD?

3. What is Katherine's gestation on the day of her first visit?

4. Compare the present fundal height with the gestation of her pregnancy. If there is a discrepancy, what are some possible causes for it?

5. What factors may have influenced Katherine to delay her first antepartum visit?

6. What factors may increase the risk for this pregnancy?

7. What diagnostic studies should the nurse anticipate at the first prenatal visit?

ANSWERS TO SELECTED QUESTIONS

Learning Activities

1. h, b, a, g, e, c, f, d
2. Refer to Figure 7-1 and the text to complete this exercise.
3. (a) 12 weeks; (b) 16 weeks; (c) 20 weeks; (d) 36 weeks
4. (a) Bluish-purple color that often extends to the vagina and labia; cause is hyperemia. (b) Cervical softening because of softening of the connective tissue. (c) Softening of the lower uterine segment. (d) Plug caused by increased secretion of mucus from cervical glands; it blocks ascent of bacteria from the vagina. (e) Mixture of cervical mucus and a small amount of blood from disruption of the mucus plug and small capillaries of cervix.
5. (a) Bluish color (as in Chadwick's sign), thickening of vaginal mucosa, prominence of rugae, heightened sexual interest. (b) Greater pliability and distensibility of vagina. (c) Increased acidic vaginal discharge that retards growth of bacteria but favors growth of *Candida albicans* (yeast).
6. (a) Progesterone maintains the endometrial layer so that the fertilized ovum can implant and relaxes the smooth muscles of the uterus, preventing contractions. It also helps prevent tissue rejection of the fetus. (b) Corpus luteum; placenta.
7. (a) Melasma, or mask of pregnancy, a pigmented area of the forehead and cheeks. (b) Areolae and nipples darken. (c) Linea nigra extends from the top of the fundus to the symphysis. Estrogen, progesterone, and melanocyte-stimulating hormone are responsible for increased pigmentation, which is more prominent in dark-skinned women.
8. Darkening of the areolae and nipples; increased breast, nipple, and areola size; nipples become more erect; Montgomery's tubercles become prominent; increased vascularity and growth of ducts, lobes, and alveoli.
9. (a) Changes in heart sounds begin between 12 and 20 weeks and end 2 to 4 weeks after birth. (b) They may include splitting of the first heart sound and a systolic murmur heard at the left sternal border. There may also be a third heart sound.
10. Lying in the supine position places the heavy uterus over the aorta and inferior vena cava, causing temporary partial occlusion of these vessels. The woman may feel faint, lightheaded, dizzy, nauseated, or agitated or become unconscious for a short time; placental blood flow may also be reduced. Prevention or treatment is to position the woman on her side or with a pillow under one hip.
11. See pp. 113-115 and Appendix A in your text to complete this chart.
12. Increased fibrinogen and clotting factors offer protection from excess blood loss but also predisposes the woman to thrombus formation.
13. The pregnant woman breathes more deeply, and airway resistance is reduced by progesterone and prostaglandins.
14. The growing uterus eventually lifts the diaphragm and reduces lung expansion. The respiratory center becomes more sensitive to carbon dioxide and the mother hyperventilates slightly.
15. Vasocongestion from estrogen's effects causes increased vascularity and edema leading to nasal stuffiness, nosebleeds, and voice changes. It can also result in ear fullness or earaches.
16. Relaxation of the lower sphincter of the esophagus allows stomach acids to move into the esophagus, causing heartburn.
17. Hypotonia prolongs emptying time of the gallbladder and allows bile to become thicker and allows the retention of cholesterol crystals.
18. Bladder tone decreases, and bladder capacity increases; the ureters, kidneys, and pelvis may dilate, and flow of urine may be partially obstructed, leading to stasis of urine.
19. Maternal absorption of calcium increases from the first trimester of pregnancy to provide for fetal needs, which are small compared with the total maternal calcium stores in the bones.
20. The fetus draws on maternal glucose, which reduces the mother's glucose levels. During the second half of pregnancy, hormones (human placental lactogen, prolactin, estrogen, progesterone, cortisol) reduce the maternal tissue sensitivity to insulin. The mother's blood glucose levels rise to make more available for the fetus. The woman normally responds by increasing insulin production.
21. See Table 7-2 to complete this exercise. Presumptive indicators are the least reliable because they are often caused by other conditions. Probable indicators are stronger evidence but still may have other causes. Positive indicators are those caused only by pregnancy.
22. (a) Placental blood flow sounds, corresponding to maternal heart rate and rhythm. (b) Umbilical cord blood flow sounds, corresponding to fetal heart rate and rhythm.
23. (a) 10 weeks; (b) 18 to 20 weeks
24. Gravida refers to the number of times a woman has been pregnant for any amount of time. Para refers to the number of pregnancies that have delivered at 20 or more weeks of gestation, regardless of the number of infants or whether the infant was born alive or stillborn.
25. (a) November 11; (b) May 9
26. Risk factors that were not apparent at previous assessments may appear later in the pregnancy.
27. Protein, glucose, ketones, bacteria

28. (a) Uterine size is larger than expected for the length of gestation. (b) Fetal movements are more numerous, which the woman who has had a previous pregnancy is more likely to notice. (c) Weight gain is greater because of greater uterine growth, increased blood volume and amniotic fluid, and presence of more than one fetus.

29. (a) A 500-mL increase in blood volume over the singleton pregnancy. (b) Cardiac workload is higher because of increased blood volume. (c) Greater diaphragm elevation increases dyspnea. (d) Greater compression of aorta and inferior vena cava causes earlier and more pronounced supine hypotension. (e) Greater ureter compression increases edema and proteinuria. (f) Pressure on bowel increases constipation.

30. See "Women Want to Know," pp. 136-137, to complete this exercise.

31. See pp. 141-144 in your text to complete this exercise. Practice how you would really say this if you were teaching a client.

Check Yourself

1, b; 2, a; 3, d; 4, b; 5, d; 6, a; 7, c; 8, a

Case Study

1. Gravida 5, para 3, abortions 1. G = 5; T = 2; P = 1; A = 1; L = 3
2. January 12
3. 18 weeks
4. Katherine's fundal height is expected at 20 weeks, and her gestation is 18 weeks by dates. It is possible that her pregnancy is more advanced than dates would indicate, she may have hydramnios, or she could be carrying more than one fetus. However, there is a margin of 3 cm in the measurements, so the fundal height may be normal.
5. The demands of her children are a probable cause for the delay in seeking prenatal care. In addition, she may feel that she does not need early prenatal care because of her past experience. She may believe that pregnancy is not an illness and it does not demand special care. Transportation and child care are other possible problems that may interfere with future visits. In addition, she may have a low income and may not have money or insurance for prenatal care.
6. Risk factors for Katherine include her age (older than 35 years), multiparity (>4 pregnancies), low prepregnancy weight, and smoking. If she is in the lower socioeconomic group, this also increases her risk. Other risk factors may be discovered during the physical examination or from the results of laboratory studies.
7. Hemoglobin and hematocrit (H & H) or complete blood count; blood typing and Rh factor with antibody screen; VDRL (Venereal Disease Research Laboratories test) or RPR (rapid plasma reagin); rubella titer; hepatitis B screen, Pap test, urinalysis (or just a screen ["dipstick"] for protein, glucose, ketones, and bacteria). An HIV (human immunodeficiency virus) screen is often offered. Other tests may be performed based on Katherine's ethnicity (e.g., for sickle cell trait), risk factors, and medical and obstetric history.

Psychosocial Adaptations to Pregnancy

Learning Activities

1. Match each term with its definition (a-h).

_____ Attachment

a. Copying the behaviors of others

_____ Bonding

b. Fetal movements felt by the mother

_____ Emotional lability

c. Preoccupation with self

_____ Infibulation

d. Strong affection between infant and significant other

_____ Introversion

e. Inward concentration

_____ Mimicry

f. Unstable mood

_____ Narcissism

g. Emotional tie of parent to infant

_____ Quickening

h. Removal of part or all of the clitoris, labia minora, and labia majora

2. List the typical maternal responses for each trimester of pregnancy.
   a. First

   b. Second

   c. Third

3. What changes occur that make the fetus seem real to the pregnant woman?

4. How might sexual interest and activity change during pregnancy? What factors may increase or decrease interest in either of the couple?

5. How does the woman's perception of the baby change during pregnancy?
   a. First trimester

   b. Second trimester

   c. Third trimester

6. What is the significance of quickening in the woman's developing relationship with her fetus?

7. How do mimicry and role play help a woman adjust to the maternal role?

8. Why might grief have a place during a desired and normal pregnancy?

9. Describe the four maternal tasks of pregnancy according to Rubin.

a.

b.

c.

d.

10. Describe the three developmental processes that the expectant father goes through during pregnancy.

a.

b.

c.

11. Describe three major factors that influence grandparents' responses to pregnancy and birth.

a.

b.

c.

12. Describe ways to ease the adaptation of siblings to the birth of an infant.
a. Toddlers

b. Preschoolers

c. School-aged children

d. Adolescents

13. How may each of these factors influence a woman's psychosocial adaptation to pregnancy?
a. Young age

b. Multiparity

c. Lack of social support

d. Absence of a partner

14. How does orientation toward the future differ among families that are affluent, middle class, working poor, and newly poor? What accounts for these differences?
a. Affluent

b. Middle class

c. Working poor

d. Newly poor

15. List barriers to prenatal care.

16. Identify types of cultural differences that can cause conflict with health care workers or interfere with a woman obtaining care.

17. What is meant by "cultural negotiation"?

Check Yourself

1. A woman who is 12 weeks pregnant begins wearing maternity clothes. This is most likely an example of
   a. Introversion
   b. Mimicry
   c. Narcissism
   d. Fantasy

2. Choose the maternal behavior that best describes role playing during pregnancy.
   a. The woman shifts from saying "I am pregnant" to "I am having a baby."
   b. The woman begins calling her fetus by a name rather than "it."
   c. The woman tries to care for infants while an experienced mother watches.
   d. The woman becomes less absorbed in her own needs and focuses on the fetus.

3. The nurse can best help a man assume his role as a parent by
   a. Encouraging him to attend prenatal visits with the woman and ask questions
   b. Referring him to prenatal discussion groups for expectant fathers
   c. Advising the woman to limit discussions of her symptoms during early pregnancy
   d. Enrolling him in childbirth classes to involve him actively in the birth

4. Choose the most likely reaction of an 8-year-old to his mother's pregnancy.
   a. Embarrassment or shame at his mother's appearance
   b. Inability to sense the reality of the infant
   c. Desire to role play his big-brother status
   d. Interest in learning about the developing baby

5. The nurse is teaching a Laotian woman about self-care during pregnancy. The nurse can best determine whether the woman has learned the information by
   a. Asking the woman to indicate what teaching she did and did not understand
   b. Observing for the woman's eye contact with the nurse during teaching
   c. Recognizing that nodding while being taught indicates understanding
   d. Having the woman restate the information that is taught

6. A pregnant woman asks the nurse whether it is safe to continue sexual intercourse during pregnancy. The nurse should tell her that intercourse
   a. Is safe if she has no complications and the membranes are intact
   b. May be rather uncomfortable after about 30 weeks of gestation
   c. Should be limited during the first and last trimesters
   d. May precipitate preterm labor if she has an orgasm

Developing Insight

1. Talk to a pregnant woman about her psychological reactions to pregnancy. Compare her reactions with typical responses listed in the text.

2. Talk with expectant fathers about when their baby first became real to them.

3. Observe interactions of the nursing staff with a woman who did not have prenatal care. Do you note any differences from the interactions with women who have had prenatal care?

4. What are the major cultural groups you encounter in the clinical setting? What specific practices or beliefs relating to pregnancy and birth can you identify that are unique to each group?

Case Study

Sara is a 17-year-old who is making her first visit to the prenatal clinic at 24 weeks of gestation with her first pregnancy. She tells you that she didn't expect to become pregnant although she did not use contraception. She has little contact with the baby's father. Sara quit school during her senior year of high school because she is embarrassed about her situation. She has gained 20 lb and feels that she is unattractive and fat. She is the oldest of six children and lives at home with her parents.

1. What factors may be involved in Sara's delay in seeking prenatal care?

2. What two priority nursing diagnoses are suggested by Sara's situation?

3. What potential conflicts are likely between Sara and the clinic staff (physicians and nurses)?

4. What services other than prenatal care is Sara likely to need because of her situation?

5. What long-term consequences are more likely because of Sara's pregnancy at this time in her life? Why?

ANSWERS TO SELECTED QUESTIONS

Learning Activities

1. d, g, f, h, e, a, c, b
2. (a) Anxiousness to determine whether pregnancy has occurred, ambivalence, focus on the self. (b) Focus on the fetus, narcissism, introversion, focus on body changes. (c) Feelings of vulnerability, fantasies or nightmares, increased dependence, desire to see the baby, worry about labor, or being anxious for the pregnancy to end.
3. Increase in uterine size, weight gain, breast changes, ultrasound images, fetal movements (quickening), hearing the fetal heartbeat
4. May be heightened or reduced. The woman may be more responsive because pelvic vasocongestion heightens sensitivity and lubricates the vaginal area. Fear of miscarriage, harming the fetus, or causing discomfort may suppress sexual desire in either partner. The woman may feel less attractive, or her partner may find her less attractive at this time. Sexuality during pregnancy may be encouraged or taboo in the couple's culture.
5. (a) The fetus seems vague and unreal, rather than seeming like a baby to her. (b) The woman perceives the fetus as real and needing her protection and has growing sense of the fetus as a separate person. (c) The woman wants to see her baby and get to know the baby as a separate being.
6. It makes the fetus seem much more like a separate being rather than a part of the woman's body.
7. They help the woman learn more about the role of a pregnant woman or a mother.
8. The woman must give up life as a carefree woman and loses spontaneity to go places and do things without planning when she becomes a mother.
9. (a) Seeking safe passage for herself and her baby. (b) Securing acceptance of herself and her baby from significant others. (c) Learning to give of herself to others. (d) Developing attachment to the unknown child.
10. (a) Grappling with reality of pregnancy and a new child. (b) Struggling for recognition as a parent. (c) Making an effort to be seen as relevant to the childbearing process.
11. (a) Age, including whether they are still working and whether they believe they are "old enough" to be grandparents. (b) Other grandchildren—excitement about the first, but less enthusiasm for subsequent grandchildren. (c) Perception of their role as grandparents—are they a source of information and support or are professionals the experts? Do they want to be very involved or less involved with grandchildren?

12. (a) Make any changes in sleeping areas before the infant arrives; prepare others for the toddler's feelings of resentment and jealousy; reassure the toddler frequently of parents' love. (b) May need help in understanding what a newborn is like and that the baby will not be a playmate; need assurance of parents' love; sibling classes are helpful. (c) Enlist their help in preparing for the baby, give information about growth and changes in the fetus; give them time alone with parents. (d) Involve them to the extent they are comfortable, because they may be embarrassed by their parents' obvious sexuality, may be preoccupied with their own issues, or may look forward to the infant.
13. (a) May have difficulty putting aside her own desires for the well-being of an infant; must give of herself before developmentally prepared to do so. (b) May grieve for the exclusive relationship with first child; concern about having enough time and energy to spread around; concern about acceptance of new infant by other child or children. (c) May need more social services, may not follow good health practices. (d) May be low-income and have late prenatal care; must enlist others to provide support that a partner would provide, may need social services such as the Special Supplemental Food Program for Women, Infants, and Children (WIC).
14. (a) Affluent families are future-oriented because their income provides security to meet their needs and prepare for their children easily. (b) Middle-class families have adequate income and work to obtain health insurance to cover medical care; they are also future-oriented. (c) Working poor families can barely meet today's needs because of low-paying jobs, so they often delay health care needs until they cannot be ignored; they may have unstable housing and food situations. (d) The newly poor are unaccustomed to such uncertainty about the future; they have future-oriented attitudes, but loss of jobs places them in need of public assistance, which they often find distressing.
15. Financial; long wait for initial visit; inability to get appointment outside of work hours; lack of transportation or child care; unsympathetic attitude of some health care workers; fear that the pregnancy will be confirmed; belief that prenatal care is unimportant.
16. Health beliefs about how to maintain health, the role of fate, illness prevention, how to restore health; modesty; female genital cutting; language differences; communication styles; eye contact; touch; and orientation to time.
17. Identification of and sensitivity to family beliefs that may differ from those of the nurse, explanation of recommendations made, compromise to find the best solution that will maintain health and the family's needs.

Check Yourself

1, b; 2, c; 3, a; 4, d; 5, d; 6, a

Case Study

1. Inadequate financial resources may have been an important reason Sara delayed prenatal care, because she has limited income of her own and may be unable to depend on her parents for money. In addition, she has no partner support and apparently feels isolated. Embarrassment and fear of her family's response, especially because she has five siblings, may also play a part. Since she did not know what to do, she may have simply done nothing.

2. Ineffective Health Maintenance and Disturbed Body Image are the priority nursing diagnoses this situation suggests. Other nursing diagnoses might include Interrupted Family Processes and Deficient Knowledge because they contribute to the priority nursing diagnoses.

3. Potential conflicts include Sara's late entry into prenatal care, possible erratic clinic visits, and possible noncompliance with professionals' recommendations.

4. Financial assistance, nutritional consultation and assistance, transportation, and other social services to help her continue her education and become self-supporting.

5. Sara is more likely to be poor because she has ended her education early. She has an increased risk of having more children soon, and her children also have a greater likelihood of ending their educations early and being poor. She is also at risk for obstetric complications. Although Sara is at higher risk for these problems, they do not have to occur. Appropriate intervention may prevent or reduce these risks.

Nutrition for Childbearing

Learning Activities

1. Match each term with its definition (a-j).

_____ Heme iron	a. Ingestion of nonfood substances
_____ Kilocalorie	b. Measure of the energy value of foods; also called calorie
_____ Lacto-ovovegetarian	c. Quality of the protein, vitamins, and minerals per 100 calories
_____ Lactovegetarian	d. Iron form most useable by body; obtained from meat, poultry, or fish
_____ Nonheme iron	e. Iron form less useable by body; obtained from plants
_____ Nutrient density	f. One who eats no animal products
_____ Ovovegetarian	g. One whose diet is primarily plant foods and who avoids animal foods
_____ Pica	h. Vegetarian who includes milk products in diet
_____ Vegan	i. Vegetarian who includes eggs in diet
_____ Vegetarian	j. Vegetarian who includes milk and eggs in diet

2. List three major consequences that are associated with inadequate prenatal weight gain.

3. List three major consequences that are associated with excessive prenatal weight gain.

4. What problems may occur when obese women become pregnant?

5. Why is the nutritional value of the diet more important than the actual weight gained during pregnancy?

6. What is the body mass index (BMI) for a woman who is 60 inches tall and weighs 145 lb?

7. List suggested pregnancy weight gains for each category.
   a. Normal prepregnancy weight (BMI 18.5 to 24.9)

   b. Prepregnancy weight underweight (BMI <18.5)

   c. Prepregnancy weight overweight (BMI 25 to 29.9)

   d. Prepregnancy weight obese (BMI >30)

8. A general guideline for pregnancy weight gain for women of normal prepregnancy weight is _____ kg (_____ lb) during the first trimester and _____ kg (_____ lb) per week thereafter.

9. Label the following figure with the appropriate weight gain for each area of the body.

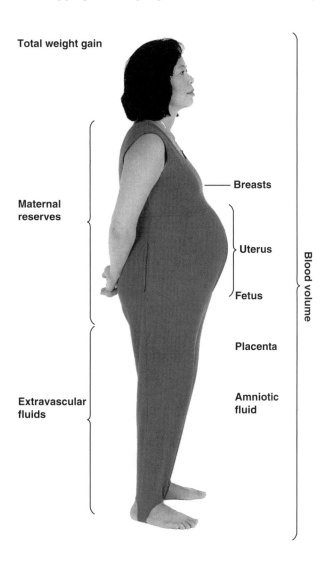

Total weight gain

Maternal reserves

Extravascular fluids

Breasts

Uterus

Fetus

Placenta

Amniotic fluid

Blood volume

10. List the calorie content for the following food types.
   a. Carbohydrates _____/g

   b. Protein _____/g

   c. Fat _____/g

11. A pregnant woman should raise her calorie consumption by _____ calories during the first trimester, _____ calories during the second trimester, and _____ calories during the third trimester. She should take in _____ calories more than her prepregnancy intake during the first 6 months of lactation and _____ more calories during the second 6 months of lactation.

12. Daily prepregnancy protein need averages _____ g. Protein need during the second half of pregnancy and for lactation is _____ g daily.

13. Name the four fat-soluble vitamins.

14. Why is folic acid important before and during pregnancy? What are some of its food sources?

15. List some high-calcium foods other than dairy foods.

16. Why might routine vitamin-mineral capsule supplementation during pregnancy cause problems?

17. The recommended fluid intake during pregnancy is _____ cups (_____ ounces) daily. Which fluids should be limited?

18. What is the recommended daily number of servings from each food group during pregnancy?
   a. Whole grains

   b. Vegetables

   c. Fruits

   d. Milk group

   e. Meat and beans group

   f. Unsaturated fats or oils

19. Explain the influence of "hot" and "cold" (or "yin" and "yang") on the diet of some pregnant women.

20. Describe the childbearing diet preferences that are typical of Southeast-Asian women.
   a. Foods encouraged during pregnancy

   b. Foods discouraged during pregnancy

   c. Postpartum changes

   d. Ways to increase nutrient intake with traditional foods

21. Describe the childbearing diet preferences that are typical of Hispanic women.
   a. Influence of "hot" and "cold" theory

   b. Common foods

   c. Common problem areas in the diet

22. Describe the following aspects of the Special Supplemental Food Program for Women, Infants, and Children (WIC).
   a. Foods provided

   b. Eligibility

23. What is the relationship between a girl's age and nutritional needs during pregnancy?

24. Describe nursing approaches that enhance the likelihood that an adolescent will follow a nutritional diet during pregnancy.

25. Explain how a vegetarian woman can meet needs of pregnancy for each nutrient listed.
   a. Protein

   b. Calcium

   c. Vitamin B$_{12}$

26. List nursing teaching that helps the pregnant woman manage nausea and vomiting.

27. What problems should the nurse watch for in the pregnant woman who has an eating disorder such as anorexia nervosa or bulimia?

28. What nutritional problems may the multipara have?

29. What additional nutritional needs does the woman with a multifetal pregnancy have?

30. What nutritional needs do women in each of these situations have?
   a. Substance abuse

   b. Smoking

   c. Alcohol abuse

31. How can each of these drugs interfere with nutrition during pregnancy?
   a. Marijuana

   b. Heroin

   c. Cocaine

   d. Amphetamine and methamphetamines

32. What problems may occur in each of these lactating mothers?
   a. Adolescent

   b. Vegan

   c. One who avoids dairy products

33. What are the recommendations for each of these substances during lactation?
   a. Alcohol

   b. Caffeine

   c. Fluid intake

34. Why is a 24-hour diet history important in counseling about nutrition?

Check Yourself

1. Calcium from green vegetables in the diet of vegans may not be used well because:
  a. They need milk to metabolize calcium adequately
  b. High iron intake interferes with calcium breakdown
  c. High fiber interferes with absorption of calcium
  d. It must be combined with a protein food

2. Poor weight gain during pregnancy is associated with
  a. Preeclampsia
  b. Congenital heart defects
  c. Preterm labor and birth
  d. Postpartum hemorrhage

3. To reduce the incidence of neural tube defects such as spina bifida, it is recommended that women of childbearing age consume
  a. 400 mcg of folic acid per day in foods and supplements
  b. 300 extra calories near the expected conception date
  c. 60 mg of supplemental iron in addition to high-iron foods
  d. 2 added servings of foods that are high in vitamin C

4. What should the nurse teach a woman about her iron supplement during pregnancy?
  a. Take the iron 30 minutes before the first food of the day.
  b. Take the iron with dairy foods to reduce the gastric side effects.
  c. Stools are somewhat loose and are lighter brown than usual.
  d. A food that is high in vitamin C may enhance absorption of iron.

5. A calcium supplement is best taken
  a. With high-iron foods
  b. At bedtime
  c. With meals
  d. On arising

6. When teaching an adolescent about nutrition during pregnancy, the nurse should
  a. Focus on the girl's responsibility to her fetus
  b. Provide as many choices as possible from nutritious foods
  c. Ask the girl to limit snacking and fast foods
  d. Explain how a good pregnancy diet will improve her health

7. The main risk to a woman who practices pica during pregnancy is
  a. Inadequate intake of essential nutrients
  b. Rapid absorption of nutrients such as iron
  c. Reduced fluid intake and dehydration
  d. Nonacceptance of the practice by caregivers

8. Choose the correct nursing approach regarding caffeine use during pregnancy.
   a. Teach that caffeine has not been shown to be a risk.
   b. Limit total intake of caffeine-containing drinks to four daily.
   c. Drink two glasses of water for each caffeine-containing drink.
   d. Discuss sources of caffeine in addition to coffee and tea.

9. A woman who is not breastfeeding is anxious to lose weight after birth. Which nursing education is most appropriate?
   a. She may begin dieting immediately because she is not breastfeeding.
   b. She should consume a minimum of 1600 calories each day to maintain energy.
   c. She should take her prenatal vitamin-mineral supplement while dieting.
   d. She should wait at least 3 weeks before beginning a diet.

Developing Insight

1. Select a cultural group that is prevalent in your clinical agency. Ask the women whether there are any foods that are encouraged or forbidden by their culture during pregnancy and the reasons for each. Ask them how long they have been in the United States and how this influences their food choices.

2. Determine what non-English diet pamphlets and teaching materials are available at your clinical facility.

3. Call your local WIC program, and tell them you are a nursing student. Ask about services they provide, eligibility criteria, and the number of women and children served in your area. If possible, observe a counseling session.

4. Complete a 24-hour diet history on yourself. Determine whether you meet the recommended number of servings for each food group and what, if any, changes you should make. What other changes would you need to make if you were pregnant?

5. Ask pregnant or postpartum women whether they have (or had) food cravings or aversions during pregnancy. What nutritional consequences might result from those you find?

Case Study

Maria is a 23-year-old Mexican-American who is pregnant with her third baby and is being seen for the first time in the clinic. Her other two children are 1 and 2 years old. Her last menstrual period was 15 weeks ago. She is 162.6 cm (64 in) tall and weighs 68.95 kg (152 lb), 6.8 kg (15 lb) more than her prepregnancy weight. Her hemoglobin is 10.3 g/dL. She says she "can't drink milk" and prefers to drink colas.

1. What is Maria's top-priority nutrition-related problem?

2. What nutritional problems are likely during this pregnancy? What foods help manage these problems?

3. What cultural aspects should the nurse consider?

ANSWERS TO SELECTED QUESTIONS

Learning Activities

1. d, b, j, h, e, c, i, a, f, g
2. Low birth weight, preterm birth, small-for-gestational-age infants, failure to begin breastfeeding
3. Macrosomia, gestational diabetes, prolonged labor, birth trauma, asphyxia, cesarean birth
4. Spontaneous abortion, gestational diabetes, preeclampsia, congenital anomalies, fetal demise, macrosomia, cesarean birth, thromboembolic disorders, and postpartum complications
5. A woman may have adequate calorie intake and gain sufficient weight yet have inadequate intake of important nutrients such as protein, iron, and folic acid. This may result in maternal anemia, inadequate fetal stores, or neural tube defects.
6. 145 lb divided by 60 inches (squared) multiplied by 703 equals 28.3. The woman is in the overweight category.
7. (a) Gain 11.5 to 16 kg (25 to 35 lb); (b) gain 12.5 to 18 kg (28 to 40 lb); (c) gain 7 to 11.5 kg (15 to 25 lb); (d) gain 5 to 9 kg (11 to 20 lb)
8. 0.5 to 2 kg (1.1 to 4.4 lb); 0.42 kg (1 lb)
9. Refer to Figure 9-1 to complete this exercise.
10. (a) 4; (b) 4; (c) 9
11. 0; 340; 452; 330; 400
12. 46; 71
13. A, D, E, and K
14. Lack of folic acid just before conception and during the early weeks of pregnancy can cause neural tube defects in the fetus. Sources include green leafy vegetables, legumes, orange juice, asparagus, spinach, and fortified cereals and pasta.
15. Legumes, nuts, dark green leafy vegetables, broccoli, dried fruit, salmon or sardines with bones, tofu
16. Excessive amounts of one vitamin or mineral may reduce absorption of others; high doses of some (e.g., vitamin A) are toxic; a false sense of security may develop that causes the woman to eat a less healthful diet.
17. 8 to 10; 64 to 80; limit carbonated drinks, coffee, tea, and high-sugar "juice" drinks
18. (a) 7 with at least one-half of the servings from whole grains; (b) 5 (2<cf>1/2 cups), with 3 cups dark green vegetables, 2 cups orange vegetables; 3 cups legumes, 3 cups starchy vegetables, and 6<cf>1/2 cups other vegetables each week; (c) 4 (2 cups); (d) 3; (e) seven 1-oz servings or two 3.5-oz servings; (f) 2 tbsp
19. Yin (cold) and yang (hot) apply to foods and conditions in many cultures, influencing what the woman eats during her pregnancy. She will balance a "hot" condition such as pregnancy by eating "cold" foods and vice versa.

20. (a) Sour foods, fruits, noodles, spinach, mung beans. (b) Fish, excessively salty or spicy foods, alcohol, rice, and unfamiliar foods. (c) "Hot" foods, such as rice with fish sauce, broth, salty meats, fish, chicken, eggs, and hot drinks. (d) Increase in dark green leafy vegetables increases calcium, iron, magnesium, folic acid; tofu or broth from vinegar-soaked pork or chicken bones increases calcium and iron; meat or poultry intake increases protein, iron, vitamin B_6 and zinc.
21. (a) Pregnancy is considered "hot," and postpartum period is considered "cold," so diet is adjusted to balance. (b) Foods include dried beans, rice, corn, tortillas, cheese, chili peppers, tomatoes, viandas, guavas, papaya, mango, and eggplant. (c) Diet is high in fiber and complex carbohydrates but also high in fat and calories (overweight is a problem).
22. (a) Milk, cheese, eggs, iron-fortified cereal, fruits and vegetables, juice, dried beans or peas, peanut butter, infant formula. (b) Income of 185% of the federal poverty level or lower; eligible throughout pregnancy and for 6 months postpartum if formula feeding or 1 year if breastfeeding.
23. Young girls who are still growing may add weight and fat to their own bodies instead of to the fetus, causing smaller infants. Maternal growth may adversely affect blood flow to the placenta and transfer of nutrients to the fetus.
24. Focus only on necessary changes; ask for the teenager's input; help her make changes that still keep her diet similar to that of her peers.
25. (a) Combine vegetable foods that have complementary amino acids within a meal or within a day, or eat small amounts of complete protein foods (e.g., cheese). (b) Calcium-fortified juices or soy products or supplement. (c) B_{12}-fortified foods or supplement.
26. Frequent small meals; reduce fatty foods; drink liquids between meals; protein snack at bedtime; carbohydrate food before getting out of bed in the morning.
27. Fears about gaining weight may resurface during pregnancy or the postpartum period. The nurse should watch for inadequate weight gain and should teach the woman the expected gain and the expected postpartum weight loss.
28. May begin pregnancy with a nutritional deficit if she has had several pregnancies (usually 5 or more), especially if they are closely spaced. Meeting nutritional and other needs of her family may take priority over her own needs.
29. She needs to eat enough to supply all the fetuses as well as meet her own needs. She needs 300 extra calories daily for each fetus and supplementation with calcium, iron, magnesium, zinc, and folic acid.
30. (a) Obtaining substance is more important than eating well, and she may lack money for food. (b) Smoking decreases appetite. Needs a vitamin-mineral supplement

because some nutrients may not be absorbed. (c) Deficient ability to absorb and use protein, niacin, vitamin B$_6$, thiamin, folic acid, magnesium, zinc; impaired metabolism; alcohol may replace food in the diet. Needs vitamin-mineral supplement.

31. (a) Increases appetite, but women may not eat foods of good quality. (b) Alters metabolism and may lead to malnutrition. (c) Appetite suppressant; vasoconstriction reduces nutrient flow to fetus; tendency to drink more alcohol or caffeine-containing beverages. (d) Depresses appetite.

32. (a) Adolescents may be deficient in many nutrients, especially iron and vitamin A. (b) The woman's milk may be low in vitamins B$_{12}$ and D. (c) Needs calcium and vitamin D from other sources.

33. (a) Avoid alcohol in general; occasional single glass of alcoholic beverage may not be harmful; larger amounts may reduce milk-ejection reflex and be harmful to infant. Avoid breastfeeding for 2 hours after drinking alcohol. (b) Limit intake to the equivalent of 2 cups of coffee; excess can make the infant irritable. (c) Drink 8 to 10 glasses or more according to thirst (excluding caffeinated beverages).

34. A 24-hour diet history helps determine the woman's usual intake, foods she likes or dislikes, and areas of deficiency.

Check Yourself

1, c; 2, c; 3, a; 4, d; 5, c; 6, b; 7, a; 8, d; 9, d

Case Study

1. Low hemoglobin (10.3 g/dl)

2. Anemia is a problem because of Maria's low hemoglobin at her initial visit and the close spacing of her children. Inadequate calcium intake is another problem because she may be lactose intolerant. Continued excess weight gain may occur because her current weight gain is 3.8 to 5.6 kg (8.6 to 12.3 lb) more than would be expected at this point in her pregnancy. Refer to Table 9-5 and Box 9-1 for food sources of iron and nondairy calcium.

3. The nurse should consider whether Maria adheres to "hot" and "cold" foods during childbearing. If Maria does not speak and read English, a fluent Spanish-speaking professional is ideal to help her understand her nutritional needs. If she reads Spanish, pamphlets in Spanish may be helpful. Maria may also need referral to the Special Supplemental Food Program for Women, Infants, and Children (WIC) if her income is low.

Antepartum Fetal Assessment

Learning Activities

1. Match each term with its definition (a-i).

_____ Alpha-fetoprotein (AFP)

_____ Amniocentesis

_____ Bilirubin

_____ Chorionic villus sampling

_____ Hydramnios

_____ Multiple-marker screen

_____ Oligohydramnios

_____ Percutaneous umbilical blood sampling

_____ Ultrasonography

a. Imaging technique that uses high-frequency sound waves to visualize internal body structures

b. Less amniotic fluid than normal

c. More amniotic fluid than normal

d. Waste product of erythrocyte (red blood cell) breakdown

e. Procedure to obtain tissue from fetal side of the developing placenta

f. Sampling fetal blood with the aid of ultrasound

g. Withdrawing amniotic fluid for laboratory examination

h. Fetal substance used to screen for specific abnormalities

i. Alpha-fetoprotein, human chorionic gonadotropin, unconjugated estriol, inhibin A

2. List typical purposes for an ultrasound examination during the
   a. First trimester

   b. Second and third trimesters

3. In which type of ultrasound examination, transvaginal or transabdominal, is a full bladder often needed? What is the reason? What effect may this have on the woman?

4. Under what circumstances is an accurate gestational age especially important? How is it assessed by ultrasonography? When is the gestational age determination most accurate?

5. What conditions are suggested by alpha-fetoprotein levels that are
   a. Low

   b. High

6. What is multiple-marker screening, and what is its purpose? What follow-up tests may be needed?

7. Chorionic villus sampling (CVS) is done between _____ and _____ weeks of pregnancy. Results are usually available in what length of time?

8. List risks of CVS.

9. List purposes for amniocentesis during the
   a. Second trimester (midtrimester)

   b. Third trimester

10. What lecithin/sphingomyelin (L/S) ratio suggests that the fetal lungs are mature? In what maternal disorder may this ratio not be associated with fetal lung maturity?

11. What is the purpose of each of the following tests from amniotic fluid? What may alter amniotic fluid tests for fetal lung maturity?
   a. Phosphatidylglycerol (PG) and phosphatidylinositol (PI)

   b. TDx assay

12. Midtrimester amniocentesis results for genetic studies are known in approximately what length of time?

13. List risks of midtrimester amniocentesis.

14. a. List indications for performing percutaneous umbilical blood sampling (PUBS).

   b. What risks are involved with percutaneous umbilical blood sampling?

15. What is the purpose of a vibroacoustic stimulation test (VAS)?

16. The basic principle of the contraction stress test is to observe the response of the _____ to the stress of _____.

17. What two methods are used to cause uterine contractions in a contraction stress test?

18. Describe possible results and implications of a contraction stress test.
a.

b.

c.

d.

e.

19. The biophysical profile assesses which fetal parameters?
a.

b.

c.

d.

e.

20. What is the significance of oligohydramnios?

Check Yourself

1. The fetal heartbeat should be visible on ultrasound by the
 a. Fourth week following the last menstrual period
 b. Sixth week following the last menstrual period
 c. Ninth week following the last menstrual period
 d. Twelfth week following the last menstrual period

2. Fewer fetal movements than expected suggest possible
 a. Intrauterine fetal growth restriction
 b. Inaccurate gestational age dating
 c. Rapid intrauterine fetal maturation
 d. Reduced placental perfusion with fetal hypoxia

3. Choose appropriate client teaching related to maternal serum alpha-fetoprotein (MSAFP) analysis.
 a. Abnormal MSAFP levels should be followed by more specific tests.
 b. High MSAFP levels are usually associated with chromosome abnormalities.
 c. Having MSAFP testing eliminates the need to do an ultrasound examination.
 d. The initial MSAFP testing will be performed at 12 weeks of gestation.

4. Choose the correct client teaching to follow amniocentesis.
 a. Drink 1 to 2 quarts of clear fluid to replace fluid taken in the procedure.
 b. Resume all normal activities when desired.
 c. Report persistent contractions, vaginal bleeding, fluid leaking, or fever.
 d. Eat a diet with increased iron for the 2 days after amniocentesis.

5. You are observing for fetal heart rate (FHR) accelerations in a nonstress test (NST) for a woman who is 26 weeks pregnant. The average FHR baseline is 145 to 155 beats per minute (bpm). Within 20 minutes, the FHR accelerated to 165 six times for 10 to 15 seconds. How should you interpret this information?
 a. Results are nonreassuring, and another 20 minutes of monitoring is needed.
 b. Results are nonreassuring because of too few accelerations within the time period.
 c. Results are reassuring because the FHR accelerated 10 bpm for 10 seconds.
 d. Results are reassuring because the fetus was inactive during the monitoring.

6. A woman who is assessing fetal movements each day should notify her health care provider if
 a. More than six movements are felt during a 30- to 60-minute period
 b. Fetal movements are fewer than the minimum set by the provider
 c. The movement pattern remains about the same from day to day
 d. Fetal movements are more frequent during the evening than in the morning

Developing Insight

1. Test your knowledge of nonstress tests. Using Figure 10-1, *A* and *B*, in the text (and reproduced here), answer the following questions about each strip.

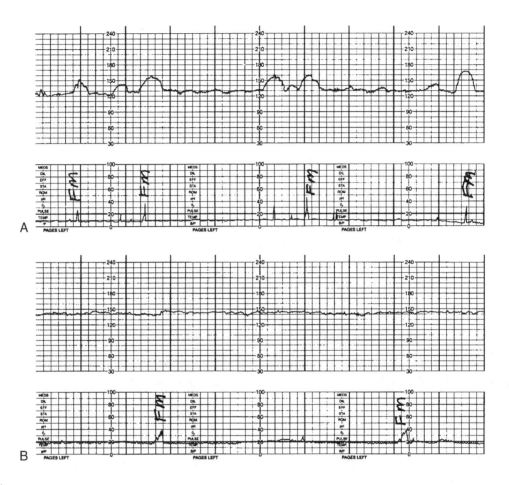

Figure 10-1, *A:*
  a. Baseline FHR?

  b. Time duration of each strip?

  c. Number of accelerations?

  d. Number of decelerations?

  e. Beats per minute and duration of the accelerations?

  f. Reactive? Why or why not?

Figure 10-1, *B:*

    a. Baseline FHR?

    b. Time duration of each strip?

    c. Number of accelerations?

    d. Number of decelerations?

    e. Beats per minute and duration of the accelerations?

    f. Reactive? Why or why not?

2. What multiple markers do you see that are offered to women you see in clinical practice? Do these women have greater risk factors for having an infant with one or more of the disorders that the screening may find?

Case Studies

Instructions: To answer the questions posed, you may need to look up information in a later chapter of your textbook so that you will understand the pathophysiology that underlies the testing.

1. Joann is a primigravida with preeclampsia in week 35 of her pregnancy. She is scheduled for amniocentesis this morning.

    a. Why is she having the test?

    b. What preprocedure and postprocedure care is indicated for any amniocentesis?

2. Betty has had type 1 diabetes for 12 years. She is beginning week 32 of her pregnancy and is scheduled for a nonstress test.

a. Why is she having the test?

b. What findings suggest that the fetus is healthy?

c. How often is this test likely to be performed?

ANSWERS TO SELECTED QUESTIONS

Learning Activities

1. h, g, d, e, c, i, b, f, a
2. (a) Confirm pregnancy and its location, gestational age, whether pregnancy is multifetal; confirm fetal viability; adjunct to chorionic villus sampling; identify fetal markers that suggest major anomalies. (b) Confirm fetal viability, gestational age and growth; locate placenta; determine fetal presentation and anatomy; evaluate amniotic fluid volume and fetal movement; adjunct to amniocentesis and percutaneous umbilical blood sampling; evaluate umbilical cord.
3. Transabdominal. Elevates the uterus and displaces the gas-filled intestines if needed. Discomfort in bladder area when scanned.
4. Accurate gestational age is needed for best maternal serum alpha-fetoprotein evaluation, to identify intrauterine growth restriction, or if there is a question about the expected date of birth. It is most accurately assessed during the first trimester by measuring the crown-rump length. During the last half of pregnancy, gestational age is assessed by several measurements, including the biparietal diameter, femur length, and abdominal circumference. From 24 to 32 weeks of gestation, two or three serial ultrasound measures taken 2 weeks apart can better establish gestational age when they are compared with standard fetal growth curves.
5. Refer to Box 10-3 on p. 204.
6. Multiple-marker screening includes maternal serum alpha-fetoprotein, human chorionic gonadotropin, unconjugated estriols, and sometimes inhibin A. Screening increases detection of trisomies, such as trisomy 18 and trisomy 21. Follow-up for abnormal levels may include amniocentesis with karyotyping.
7. 10; 12; preliminary results in 2 to 3 hours; 2 to 4 days for improved quality of test results; 7 days for tissue culture analysis; varying time of results for tests other than karyotyping
8. Pregnancy loss, infection, limb reduction defects, Rh sensitization, expense, unexpected need for added tests
9. (a) Refer to Box 10-4 on p. 207 to answer this question. (b) Evaluate fetal lung maturity, identify fetal hemolytic disease
10. Ratio of 2:1; diabetes mellitus
11. (a) Presence in the amniotic fluid confirms fetal lung maturity. (b) Determines surfactant content in amniotic fluid. All tests may be affected by the presence of blood or meconium in the fluid.
12. Three to seven days for chromosome analysis, depending on the test. More rapid results may include analysis using DNA probes, fluorescent probes (fluorescent in-situ hybridization [FISH]), or spectral karyotyping. Time required to test for specific disorders varies.
13. Pregnancy loss, fetal hemorrhage if the placenta or cord is pierced, Rh sensitization
14. (a) Management of Rh disease; genetic studies; diagnosis of abnormal fetal blood clotting factors; treatment of fetal blood diseases or delivery of therapeutic drugs that cannot be delivered to the fetus in another way. (b) Bradycardia, prolonged bleeding, cord laceration, cord hematoma, thrombosis, thromboembolism, preterm labor, preterm rupture of membranes, maternal blood sensitization.
15. VAS identifies whether fetal heart rate (FHR) accelerations occur in response to sound stimulation; it shortens nonstress test (NST) or confirms a nonreactive NST. VAS can be used in the intrapartum period to clarify questionable findings.
16. FHR; uterine contractions
17. Breast self-stimulation, oxytocin infusion
18. (In any order) (a) Negative (reassuring)–no late decelerations (decreases in the FHR that persist after the contraction ends) occurred in the FHR, although the fetus was stressed by three contractions of at least 40 seconds duration in a 10-minute period; (b) Positive (abnormal)–50% or more of contractions are accompanied by late decelerations, even if there are fewer than three contractions in 10 minutes; (c) Equivocal (suspicious)– intermittent late FHR decelerations and significant variable decelerations; (d) Equivocal (tachysystole)–FHR decelerations that occur in the presence of contractions that are closer than every 2 minutes or last longer than 90 seconds; (e) Unsatisfactory–fewer than three contractions in 10 minutes or any tracing that cannot be interpreted.
19. (In any order) (a) FHR activity as in the NST; (b) fetal breathing movements; (c) gross fetal movements; (d) fetal tone; (e) amniotic fluid volume
20. During fetal hypoxemia, blood is shunted away from the kidneys and lungs and toward the brain, resulting in a lower amniotic fluid volume. It may indicate chronic fetal hypoxia.

Check Yourself

1, b; 2, d; 3, a; 4, c; 5, c; 6, b

Developing Insight

1. Figure 10-1, *A:* (a) 125 to 130 bpm; (b) 10 minutes; (c) seven total, four occurring with marked fetal movement (FM); (d) none; (e) 25 to 30 bpm; duration 20 to 30 seconds; (f) reactive: in this 10-minute period, there are at least two accelerations peaking at 15 bpm or more and that have a duration of at least 15 seconds

Figure 10-1, *B:* (a) 140 to 145 bpm; (b) 10 minutes; (c) none; (d) none; (e) no accelerations to analyze; (f) the test is incomplete because less than 20 minutes have elapsed; however, if there are still no accelerations during the next 30 minutes, the test will be nonreactive; this strip could have caught the fetus in a sleep cycle

Case Studies

1. (a) Pregnancy-induced hypertension may reduce placental perfusion, and delivery of the baby is its only real cure. The amniocentesis is most likely being performed to assess fetal lung maturity. If the lungs are mature, induction of labor is likely. (b) Preamniocentesis care: Displacement of uterus with a rolled towel under the hip; assessment of maternal blood pressure and FHRs; ultrasound location of fetus, placenta, and largest pockets of amniotic fluid. Postamniocentesis care: maternal rest with electronic fetal monitoring; caution to avoid strenuous activity for 1 or 2 days; teach to report uterine contractions, vaginal bleeding, leaking amniotic fluid, fever.

2. (a) Diabetes is a disorder involving the blood vessels, and there is a possibility that the placental function is impaired because of this maternal condition. (b) Findings that suggest normal placental function through the NST include a normal baseline FHR with long-term variability of at least 10 bpm and two or more FHR accelerations of at least 15 bpm for at least 15 seconds within a 20-minute time period, with or without fetal movement. (c) The test will probably be repeated at least weekly.

Perinatal Education

Learning Activities

1. Match each term with its definition (a-h).

_____ Birth plan

_____ Bradley method

_____ Dick-Read method

_____ Doula

_____ Effleurage

_____ Habituation

_____ Lamaze method

_____ Leboyer childbirth

a. First called "natural childbirth"

b. Sometimes referred to as "birth without violence"

c. Often called the "psychoprophylaxis" method of childbirth

d. Identifies preferences for the birth experience

e. Called "husband-coached childbirth"

f. Decreased response to repeated stimulus

g. Massage on abdomen during contractions

h. A person hired to provide support during labor or in the postpartum period

2. What does each of these factors have to do with a woman's choice to take childbirth classes?
   a. Income

   b. Desire to participate

   c. Fear

3. What are some choices a woman must make regarding childbearing?

4. List content typically covered in early pregnancy classes.
   a. Preconception classes

   b. First trimester

   c. Second trimester

5. List three important precautions for exercise classes during pregnancy.
   a.

   b.

   c.

6. What are important topics to discuss related to cesarean birth preparation in each type of class?
   a. General childbirth class

   b. Planned cesarean birth class

7. Describe the importance of each factor in managing birth pain.

a. Education

b. Relaxation

c. Conditioning

8. List the basic characteristics of each variation of childbirth education.

a. Dick-Read

b. Bradley

c. Leboyer

d. Lamaze

9. Explain how each of these techniques can help the woman during childbirth.

a. Relaxation

b. Cutaneous stimulation

c. Effleurage

d. Sacral pressure

e. Thermal stimulation

f. Mental stimulation

    g. Focal point

    h. Imagery

    i. Music

    j. Hydrotherapy

10. What variations in the role of support person is the nurse likely to encounter?

11. Describe techniques the labor partner may use in each area.
    a. Monitoring the contraction pattern

    b. Environmental management

    c. Comfort measures

Check Yourself

1. A primary benefit of a preconception class is to
    a. Reduce the risk of having a baby with a birth defect
    b. Begin the pregnancy in an optimal health state
    c. Limit the number of unplanned pregnancies in the community
    d. Encourage the couple to have their baby at that facility

2. Firm pressure on the palms may reduce labor pain because it
    a. Stimulates large-diameter nerve fibers, interfering with transmission of pain
    b. Provides a focal point on a body part other than the uterus or vaginal area
    c. Avoids habituation to repeated stimuli, thus enhancing pain relief
    d. Allows the woman to relax body parts other than her hands

3. The primary benefit of perinatal education is to help
   a. Reduce the likelihood that parents will have problems with their infant
   b. Women have a satisfying childbirth free of medication or other interventions
   c. Parents become active in health maintenance during pregnancy and birth
   d. Enhance the chance that prospective parents will return to the hospital

4. A man accompanies his wife during her labor with her first baby. He stays nearby but does not take an active role. The nurse should
   a. Ask the couple whether there is a support person who can better support the woman
   b. Perform all coaching needed by the woman during her labor and birth
   c. Assume that his cultural role does not permit him to take an active part in labor
   d. Offer to teach him simple techniques that he may use to help his wife give birth

5. The purpose of a birth plan is to help the woman or couple
   a. Choose which medications the woman will use
   b. Decide whether they want intravenous (IV) lines, monitors, and the like
   c. Have a basis for communicating with caregivers
   d. Avoid the need for a cesarean birth

Developing Insight

1. With a partner, practice each specific relaxation technique. What is the benefit of each?
   a. Progressive relaxation

   b. Neuromuscular dissociation

   c. Touch relaxation

   d. Relaxation against pain

2. Based on the knowledge you have gained, prepare a birth plan that you would like, identifying any special preferences you would like to include in a birth experience.

3. Attend a class on preparing for childbirth. Compare what couples learn about various subjects with what you learn in your classes.

4. Attend a class for siblings. Determine how you can incorporate what is taught in the classes in your teaching to help parents prepare their children for the birth of another child.

ANSWERS TO SELECTED QUESTIONS

Learning Activities

1. d, e, a, h, g, f, c, b
2. (a) Low-income women may not be able to pay for classes; they may enter prenatal care late or may have no prenatal care, or they may miss opportunities even for free classes, or may not have transportation to classes. (b) Some want education so that they can participate fully in all decisions related to childbearing. (c) Some want to obtain skills to help them cope with their fears about pain and the demands of birth.
3. A woman must decide what type of health care professional she will have, where she will give birth, who will be with her, interventions she will use during birth, and what kinds of classes she will attend, if any.
4. (a) Nutrition, pregnancy signs, healthy lifestyle, choosing a caregiver, importance of prenatal care, reducing risk factors, effects of pregnancy on relationships. (b) Dealing with discomforts common in early pregnancy, sexuality, what to expect, value of prenatal care, avoiding hazards. (c) Body mechanics, fetal development, working during pregnancy, childbirth choices, postbirth needs of mother and infant.
5. (a) Warm-up exercises; (b) low-impact activities; (c) avoiding excessive heart rate elevation
6. (a) Incidence, indications, advantages and risks of elective cesarean birth, options, surgical procedure, postoperative course. (b) Share experiences and feelings; clarify misconceptions, indications, care to expect, ways to participate more fully.
7. (a) Increases confidence, gives a chance to rehearse and practice coping techniques. (b) Enhances ability to labor efficiently and with less pain; improved use of all other pain management techniques. (c) Helps the woman respond to pain with a conditioned response of relaxation.
8. (a) Fear results in tension, which results in pain. Education and relaxation can reduce fear and therefore pain. (b) The husband is the coach; abdominal breathing and breath control are used; the woman avoids medications. (c) Philosophy is "birth without violence"; views birth as traumatic to infant; lights are dimmed, infant is given a warm bath right after birth. (d) Lamaze uses mental techniques to prevent pain, including conditioned responses to contractions with breathing and relaxation techniques.
9. (a) Conserves energy, decreases use of oxygen, and enhances other pain management techniques. (b) Stimulates large-diameter sensory nerve fibers and interferes with transmission of pain impulses to the brain by way of small-diameter fibers. (c) Increases concentration and interferes with pain impulse transmission. (d) Relieves strain on sacroiliac joint. (e) Stimulates thermoreceptors and may reduce pain sensation. (f) Increases mental concentration and interferes with pain impulses. (g) Directs thoughts away from contraction. (h) Enhances relaxation with pleasant thoughts. (i) Increases relaxation and helps pace breathing, blocks out other noise. (j) Enhances relaxation, reducing muscle tension and pressure on the abdomen.
10. Some labor partners take an active role, being involved in all aspects of birth. Some feel helpless and look to others to support the woman or to tell them how to be helpful. Some believe that men should be present but should not actively participate. Their presence alone offers a form of support.
11. (a) Alerting the mother to oncoming contraction to prepare for breathing, telling her when contraction peak has passed. (b) Turning down lights, suggesting use of music or other distractions. (c) Offering ice chips, wiping the mother's face with a cool cloth, using cold or warm packs, helping with position changes, applying sacral pressure or back rubs, giving positive feedback, coaching in learned breathing techniques.

Check Yourself

1, b; 2, a; 3, c; 4, d; 5, c

CHAPTER 12

Processes of Birth

Learning Activities

1. Match each term with its definition (a-h).

_____ Afterpains

_____ Catecholamines

_____ Dilation

_____ Effacement

_____ Molding

_____ Physiologic retraction ring

_____ Relaxin

_____ Station

a. Measurement of descent of the fetal presenting part into the pelvis

b. Opening of the cervix

c. Thinning of the cervix

d. Hormone that causes cartilage to soften

e. Change in the shape of the fetal head during birth

f. Maternal substances secreted in response to stress

g. Division between the upper and lower uterine segments

h. Postbirth uterine contractions

2. Explain why each characteristic of uterine contractions is important during birth.
   a. Coordinated

   b. Involuntary

   c. Intermittent

3. Describe differences in how the upper and lower parts of the uterus contract during labor. Why is it important that the parts have different contraction characteristics?

4. Why should the nurse regularly check the woman's bladder at the following times?
   a. During labor

   b. During the early postpartum period

5. What maternal and fetal conditions can reduce fetal tolerance for the intermittent interruption in placental blood flow that occurs during contractions?

6. What are the changes in fetal lung fluid during pregnancy and labor and after birth?

7. What are the two powers of labor? When during labor do they come into play?

8. Why are the sutures and fontanels of the fetal head important during birth?

9. Describe the most common variations in
   a. Fetal lie

   b. Fetal attitude

   c. Fetal presentation

10. Draw the three variations of a breech presentation. Which one is most common?

11. What fetal anatomic reference point is used for each presentation or position when stating fetal position?
   a. Vertex

   b. Face

   c. Breech

12. How can nursing measures help increase a woman's sense of control during labor?

13. How does each of these factors affect the onset of labor?
a. Fetal hormone production

b. Change in maternal progesterone and estrogen relationship

c. Oxytocin receptors

14. Describe common premonitory signs of labor. Note any differences between a nullipara and a parous woman.

15. Describe each mechanism of labor and its significance.
a. Descent

b. Engagement

c. Flexion

d. Internal rotation

e. Extension

f. External rotation

g. Expulsion

16. Why must the fetal head and shoulders undergo rotation within the pelvis?

17. What are the three labor phases within stage I? What cervical dilation marks each phase?
   a.

   b.

   c.

18. How does average duration of labor vary between nulliparas and parous women for active phase first and second stages of labor?

19. List four signs that suggest that the placenta has separated.
   a.

   b.

   c.

   d.

20. Why is it important that the uterus remain firmly contracted after birth?

21. Complete the following chart about the characteristics of normal labor.

	First Stage	*Second Stage*	*Third Stage*	*Fourth Stage*
Duration Nullipara				
Multipara				
Cervical dilation Latent phase				
Active phase				
Transition phase				

	First Stage	Second Stage	Third Stage	Fourth Stage
Uterine contractions Latent phase				
Active phase				
Transition phase				
Discomfort				
Maternal behaviors				

Labeling

1. Label each part of the contraction cycle.
   a. Increment
   b. Peak (acme)
   c. Decrement
   d. Frequency
   e. Duration
   f. Intensity
   g. Interval

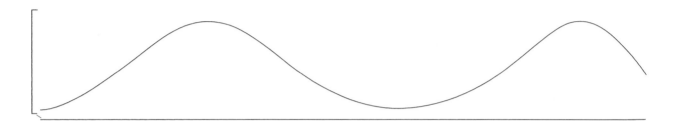

2. Label the bones, fontanels, and diameters of the fetal skull. Fill in the blanks with the normal diameters as indicated. Which anterior-posterior diameter is most favorable for vaginal birth? Some letters may be used twice.
   a. Frontal suture
   b. Lambdoid suture
   c. Coronal suture
   d. Sagittal suture
   e. Anterior fontanel
   f. Posterior fontanel
   g. Frontal bone
   h. Parietal bone
   i. Occipital bone
   j. Biparietal diameter (_____ cm)
   k. Occipitofrontal diameter (_____ cm)
   l. Suboccipitobregmatic diameter (_____ cm)
   m. Submentobregmatic diameter (_____ cm)
   n. Supraoccipitomental diameter (_____ cm)

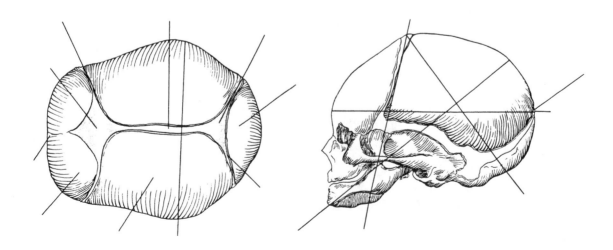

3. Label each fetal presentation and position. Circle the one that is most favorable for vaginal birth. Mark an X over the one that is least favorable.

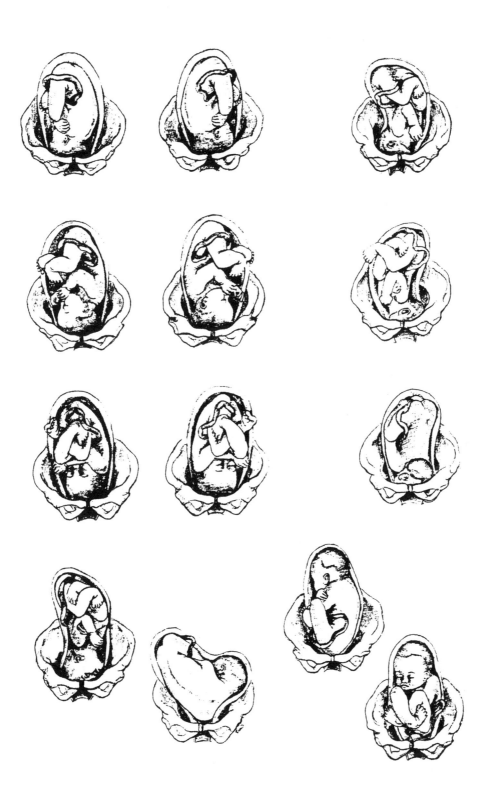

Check Yourself

1. When assessing a laboring woman's blood pressure, the nurse should
   a. Inflate the cuff at the beginning of a contraction
   b. Check the blood pressure between two contractions
   c. Expect a slight elevation of the blood pressure
   d. Position the woman on her back with her knees bent

2. A woman is admitted in active labor. Her leukocyte count is 14,500. Based on this information, the nurse should
   a. Assess the woman for other evidence of infection
   b. Inform the nurse-midwife of the results promptly
   c. Use isolation techniques to limit spread of infection
   d. Record the expected results in the woman's chart

3. The most appropriate time for the nurse to assist a laboring woman to push is
   a. During the interval between contractions
   b. During first-stage labor
   c. During second-stage labor
   d. Whenever she feels the need

4. The abbreviation LOA means that the fetal occiput is
   a. On the examiner's left and in the front of the pelvis
   b. In the left front part of the mother's pelvis
   c. Anterior to the fetal breech
   d. Lower than the fetal breech

5. Choose the most reliable evidence that true labor has begun.
   a. Regular contractions that occur every 15 minutes
   b. Change in the amount of cervical thinning
   c. Increased ease of breathing with frequent urination
   d. A sudden urge to do household tasks

6. The nurse should note how long the interval between contractions lasts because
   a. Maternal cells restore their glucose levels during the interval
   b. A very short interval requires earlier administration of analgesia
   c. Most exchange of fetal oxygen and waste products occurs then
   d. The interval becomes longer as cervical dilation increases

7. What is the primary benefit of the stress of labor to the newborn?
   a. It stimulates breathing and elimination of lung fluid.
   b. It increases alertness and enhances parent-infant bonding.
   c. It speeds peristalsis to eliminate meconium quickly.
   d. It enhances tolerance of microorganisms from others.

8. Choose the abbreviation that represents the fetal presentation and position that is most favorable for vaginal birth.
   a. LOA
   b. RMP
   c. LST
   d. ROP

9. A station of +1 means that the
   a. Maternal cervix is open 1 cm
   b. Mother's ischial spines project into her pelvis 1 cm
   c. Fetus is unlikely to be born vaginally because the pelvis is small
   d. Fetal presenting part is 1 cm below the mother's ischial spines

Developing Insight

1. Place a tennis ball in a sock. Slowly push it out of the cuff to get the idea of cervical effacement and dilation.

2. In performing a vaginal examination during labor, the nurse collects the following information.
   a. Cervix is open 4 cm, and its length is approximately 0.5 cm.
   b. The presenting part is rounded and hard. A triangular depression on the presenting part has three linear depressions leading from it. Clear fluid flows from the vagina as the fetus moves during the examination. What is the correct interpretation of these findings?

3. Which presentation is represented in the following drawing? Draw the main anterior-posterior diameter that is presenting. What landmarks on the fetal head would the nurse feel on vaginal examination? What is the likely outcome?

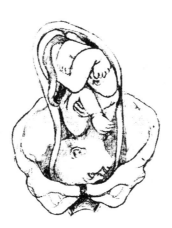

ANSWERS TO SELECTED QUESTIONS

Learning Activities

1. h, f, b, c, e, g, d, a
2. (a) Contractions must be stronger in the upper uterus than in the lower uterus to propel the fetus toward the outside. (b) Woman cannot consciously cause labor to start or stop; otherwise, many infants would be born early because the woman became tired of being pregnant, or labor might be suspended when it became intense. (c) Intervals between contractions allow resumption of blood flow to the placenta to supply oxygen and remove wastes for the fetus.
3. The upper uterus contracts actively to push the fetus downward, whereas the lower uterus is more passive to reduce resistance to fetal passage. Any other pattern would be ineffective at pushing the fetus out.
4. (a) A full bladder increases pain and interferes with fetal descent. (b) A full bladder interferes with the uterine contractions that compress open vessels to control bleeding.
5. Any maternal condition that reduces perfusion of the placenta, such as diabetes, hypertension, or fetal anemia, which reduces oxygen-carrying capacity, can reduce tolerance for even normal labor contractions.
6. In late pregnancy, production of fetal lung fluid decreases and absorption into the interstitium of the lungs increases. During labor, absorption of lung fluid intensifies and compression of the head and thorax causes expulsion of additional fluid. After birth, the remainder is absorbed into the newborn pulmonary and lymphatic circulations.
7. Uterine contractions, first stage; uterine contractions and maternal pushing, second stage
8. They allow molding to let the fetal head adapt to the size and shape of the maternal pelvis.
9. (a) Longitudinal (common) or transverse (rare); oblique lie is at some angle to a longitudinal or transverse lie; (b) flexion (common) or extension (uncommon); (c) cephalic (common), breech (approximately 3%), or shoulder (rare, less than 0.2%)
10. Refer to Figure 12-9 on p. 246 to complete this exercise. Frank breech is most common.
11. (a) Occiput; (b) chin (mentum); (c) sacrum
12. They promote relaxation and ability to work with her body's efforts rather than working against the natural forces.
13. (a) The fetus appears to secrete oxytocin and cortisol, hormones that stimulate uterine contractions. The fetal membranes also release prostaglandins during labor. (b) Higher estrogen levels make the uterus more sensitive to substances that stimulate it to contract, whereas lower progesterone levels allow it to be stimulated more easily; estrogen also increases the number of gap junctions, connections that allow the uterus to contract in a coordinated manner. (c) Oxytocin receptors increase as labor begins, continue to increase during labor, and peak at delivery.
14. Braxton Hicks contractions: irregular, mild contractions intensify near term; more noticeable to parous women. Lightening: descent of fetus toward pelvic inlet increases pressure on bladder but allows easier breathing; more noticeable in nulliparas. Increased vaginal secretions: with congestion of vaginal mucosa caused by fetal pressure. Bloody show: mixture of cervical mucus and blood as the mucus plug is released; seen earlier and in greater quantity in nulliparas. Energy spurt: Nesting. Weight loss: 2.2 to 6.6 kg (1 to 3 lb).
15. Refer to Figure 12-12 on p. 253-254 to complete this exercise.
16. The fetal head begins descent with the sagittal suture oriented in a transverse (crosswise) or oblique orientation to the woman's pelvis. As the head descends, it rotates so that the head is oriented with the sagittal suture in an anterior-posterior (OA) orientation to the woman's pelvis. After the fetal head is born, the fetal shoulders are then transverse in the pelvis and must rotate to pass under the pubic arch and be born.
17. (a) Latent phase: up to 3 cm dilation; (b) active phase: 4 to 7 cm; (c) transition phase: 8 to 10 cm
18. First stage: nullipara, 8 to 10 hours (range 6 to 18 hours); parous woman, 6 to 7 hours (range 2 to 10 hours). Second stage: nullipara, 50 minutes (range 30 minutes to 3 hours); parous woman, 20 minutes (range 5 to 30 minutes).
19. (In any order) (a) Uterus has spheric shape; (b) uterus rises upward in abdomen; (c) cord descends further from vagina; (d) gush of blood
20. Firm uterine contraction compresses bleeding vessels at the placental site to prevent hemorrhage.
21. Refer to Table 12-1 on p. 255 to complete this question.

Labeling

1. Refer to Figure 12-1 on p. 238.
2. Refer to Figure 12-5 on p. 244.
   The suboccipitobregmatic diameter, with the fetal head fully flexed, is most favorable for vaginal birth. It measures approximately 9.5 cm.
3. Refer to Figure 12-11 on p. 248.

Check Yourself

1, b; 2, d; 3, c; 4, b; 5, b; 6, c; 7, a; 8, a; 9, d

Developing Insight

2. (a) Cervical dilation is 4 cm; effacement is 75%. (b) Presentation is cephalic; membranes are ruptured, and the fluid is normal. The woman is beginning the active phase of first-stage labor.

3. The nurse would feel the fetal brow, possibly the bridge of the nose, and the anterior fontanel (diamond shaped, with four suture lines leading into it). The fetal head is likely to either flex into a vertex presentation or extend into a face presentation.

Nursing Care during Labor and Birth

Learning Activities

1. Match each term with its definition (a-e).

_____ Crowning

_____ Ferning

_____ Funic souffle

_____ pH test

_____ Uterine souffle

a. Paper or swab used to detect ruptured membranes

b. Sound of blood going through the uterine blood vessels

c. Sound of blood going through the umbilical cord

d. Appearance of the fetal presenting part at the vaginal opening

e. Characteristic appearance of dry amniotic fluid when viewed under a microscope

2. List the two nursing priority determinations when a woman enters a birth center.

a.

b.

3. Describe characteristics of the fetal heart rate (FHR) that are reassuring when the FHR is auscultated in a term fetus.

4. When should the nurse *not* perform a vaginal examination at a woman's admission? Why?

5. List important nursing assessments after the membranes rupture. Describe normal and abnormal assessment results.

6. Why is it important to place a small pillow under one hip if the mother must lie briefly on her back?

7. Describe how contractions feel to the nurse when palpated if they are
   a. Mild

   b. Moderate

   c. Strong

8. List three characteristics of tetanic (hypertonic) contractions. Why is it important to watch for this type of contraction?
   a.

   b.

   c.

9. Why is a woman's previous adverse reaction to dental anesthesia relevant to birth?

10. What maternal vital signs may indicate problems?
   a. Blood pressure

   b. Temperature

11. Describe basic comfort measures the nurse can provide during labor. Add any that you found helpful to a laboring woman during your intrapartum clinical.

Labeling

1. Describe each of Leopold's maneuvers below the four illustrations. Problem solving: How would these 4 illustrations look different for ROA presentation (problem a) and LST presentation (problem b)? What did you palpate on any of your clinical patients if you or the nurse did Leopold's? Would illustrations look like these if you drew what you felt in the clinical setting?
   a. ROA, station +1
   b. LST, station −2

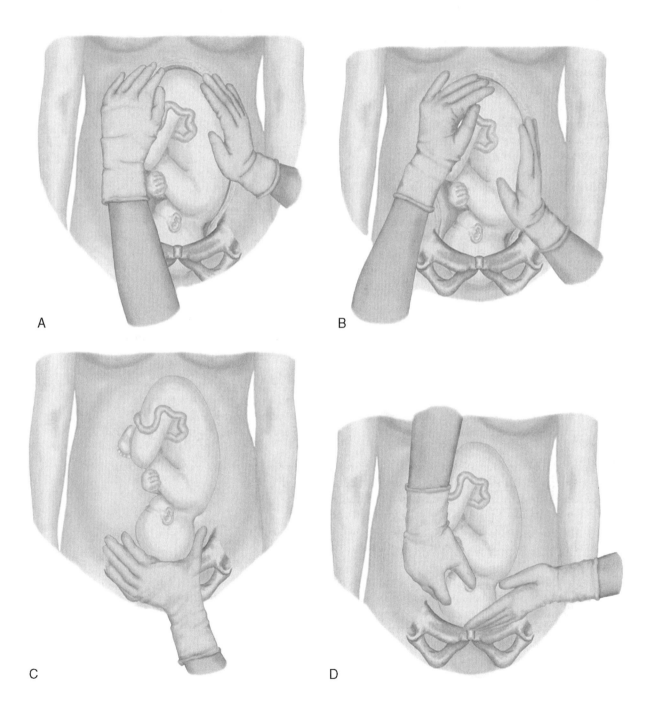

A

B

C

D

Check Yourself

1. Bloody show differs from active vaginal bleeding in that bloody show
   a. Quickly clots on the perineal pad
   b. Is dark red and mixed with mucus
   c. Flows freely during vaginal examination
   d. Decreases in quantity as labor progresses

2. A laboring woman who has not taken pain medication abruptly stops her previous breathing techniques during a contraction and makes low-pitched grunting sounds. The priority nursing action is to
   a. Ask her whether she needs pain medication
   b. Turn her to her left side
   c. Assess contraction duration
   d. Look at her perineum

3. A woman's membranes rupture during a contraction. The priority nursing action is to
   a. Assess the fetal heart rate
   b. Note the color of the discharge
   c. Check the woman's vital signs
   d. Determine whether the fluid has a foul odor

4. When palpating labor contractions, the nurse should
   a. Use the palm of one hand while palpating the lower uterus
   b. Avoid palpating during the period of maximum intensity
   c. Place the fingertips over the fundus of the uterus
   d. Limit palpation to three consecutive contractions

5. When performing Leopold's maneuvers, the nurse palpates a hard, round object in the uterine fundus. A smooth, rounded surface is on the mother's right side, and irregular movable parts are felt on her left side. An irregularly shaped fetal part is felt in the suprapubic area and is easily moved upward. How should these findings be interpreted?
   a. The fetal presentation is cephalic, position is ROA, and the presenting part is engaged.
   b. The fetal presentation is cephalic, position is LOP, and the presenting part is not engaged.
   c. The fetal presentation is breech, position is RST, and the presenting part is engaged.
   d. The fetal presentation is breech, position is RSA, and the presenting part is not engaged.

6. When performing the fourth Leopold's maneuver, the nurse determines that the cephalic prominence is on the same side as the fetal back. How should this assessment be interpreted?
   a. The fetus is in a breech presentation with the head extended.
   b. The fetus is in a face presentation with the head extended.
   c. The fetus is in a transverse lie with the face toward the mother's back.
   d. The fetus is in a cephalic presentation with the head well flexed.

7. When auscultating the fetal heart rate of a term fetus during labor, the nurse notes a rate of 130 to 140 beats per minute (bpm), with occasional accelerations in the rate. How should the nurse interpret the data?
   a. The baseline rate is slightly high for a term fetus.
   b. Accelerations in the rate suggest intermittent hypoxia.
   c. Labor usually causes the fetal heart rate to be slower.
   d. These assessments are normal for a term fetus during labor.

8. The nurse notes the following contraction pattern.

Beginning of Contraction	End of Contraction
11:15:00	11:15:40
11:20:00	11:20:45
11:24:00	11:24:50
11:28:30	11:29:10
11:33:00	11:33:35

Choose the correct documentation for the pattern.
a. Contractions every 4 to 5 minutes; duration 35 to 50 seconds
b. Contractions every 5 minutes; duration 35 to 40 seconds
c. Contractions every 3 to 5 minutes; duration 30 to 50 seconds
d. Contractions every 3 to 4 minutes; duration 30 to 40 seconds

9. A woman having her third baby planned epidural analgesia for labor and birth. However, her labor was so rapid that she did not have the epidural. What is the best initial nursing approach in this case?
a. Congratulate her on having a labor that was quicker than expected.
b. Use open-ended questions to clarify her true feelings about the experience.
c. Tactfully explain why a nonepidural labor and birth are actually better.
d. Explain that it is often difficult to time epidural analgesia for labor.

10. A woman having her first baby has been observed for 2 hours for labor but is having false labor contractions. Choose the most appropriate teaching before she returns home.
a. "It is unlikely that your labor will be fast, so you can stay home until your water breaks."
b. "If your water breaks, you can wait until contractions are 5 minutes apart or closer."
c. "As long as the baby is active, there is no hurry to return to the birth center."
d. "Your contractions will usually be 5 minutes apart or closer for 1 hour if labor is real."

Developing Insight

1. During your clinical experience, note what effects fetal presentation and position have on the woman's comfort and the progress of labor.

2. Review the routine permits obtained in the intrapartum area at your birth facility.

3. During your clinical experience, use Leopold's maneuvers to identify fetal presentation, position, and engagement. Use the previous labeling activity to identify the locations and positions of fetal parts.

Case Study

Erin is an 18-year-old primigravida who calls the intrapartum unit because she thinks she may be in labor.

1. What information should the nurse obtain to help determine whether Erin is in true labor?

The nurse decides that Erin may be in true labor and tells her to come to the birth center. On arrival, Erin says she thinks her "water broke."

2. What is the priority nursing care at this time?

3. What tests might the nurse use to verify that Erin's membranes have indeed ruptured?

The nurse determines that Erin's contractions are every 5 minutes, are of moderate intensity, and last 40 seconds. The fetus is active during the initial assessment. Fetal heart rate is 135 to 150 bpm, and the rate often accelerates. Amniotic fluid is light green with small white flecks in it. Vaginal examination reveals that the cervix is dilated 5 cm and is completely effaced. The fetal presenting part is hard and round, and a small triangular depression on the head can be felt in Erin's right posterior pelvis.

4. What stage (and phase, if applicable) of labor is Erin in?

5. How should the fetal heart rate be interpreted?

6. Is the amniotic fluid normal?

7. What is the fetal presentation and position?

Erin complains of back discomfort during each contraction.

8. What interventions might make this discomfort more tolerable?

After 4 hours of labor in the birth center, Erin's cervix is completely dilated and effaced, and the fetal station is +1. Erin feels the need to push during some contractions.

9. What is the safest way to advise Erin to push?

10. When should Erin be positioned for birth?

Erin gives birth to a boy. The nurse notes the following on the baby at 1 minute: heart rate 138 bpm; loud, vigorous crying; spontaneous movement and flexion of the extremities; and pink skin color except for bluish color of the hands and feet.

11. What Apgar score will be assigned to the baby?

12. What are the priority nursing measures for the infant in relation to
   a. Respiration

   b. Temperature regulation

Erin is now in the fourth stage of labor. She and her husband are getting acquainted with their baby, Derrick.

13. What time period does the fourth stage involve?

14. What nursing assessments are needed to observe for hemorrhage?

15. What are appropriate pain-relief methods during the fourth stage?

ANSWERS TO SELECTED QUESTIONS

Learning Activities

1. d, e, c, a, b
2. (a) Condition of the mother and fetus; (b) nearness to birth
3. Heart rate at term with a lower limit of 110 beats per minute (bpm), upper limit of 160 bpm; regular rhythm; presence of accelerations; absence of decelerations. These signs would also be reassuring if the fetus were monitored electronically. (See Chapter 14 for added information about the electronically monitored fetus.)
4. Vaginal examination should not be routinely performed (a) if the woman is bleeding actively, because the examination may increase bleeding; bloody show is not a contraindication to vaginal examination; (b) if fetal gestation is ≤36 weeks because of stimulation of preterm labor or preterm membrane rupture (see also Chapter 27).
5. Time of rupture; whether rupture was spontaneous or artificial; quantity of fluid; fetal heart rate (FHR) for at least 1 minute; color of fluid (clear, possibly with bits of vernix, is normal; green indicates fetal meconium passage; yellow or cloudy suggests infection); odor (foul or strong odor suggests infection)
6. To prevent supine hypotension from aortocaval compression by the heavy uterus
7. (a) Uterus is easily indented; like the tip of the nose. (b) Can be indented, but with more difficulty; like the chin. (c) Little indentation is possible; "woody" feel; like the forehead.
8. (In any order) (a) Durations longer than 90 to 120 seconds; (b) intervals shorter than 30 seconds; (c) incomplete uterine relaxation between contractions. If tetanic, or hypertonic, contractions are too long or too frequent, or if too little uterine relaxation exists, fetal oxygenation may be reduced.
9. Dental anesthesia is related to many of the local anesthetic agents used in regional and local anesthetics such as epidurals.
10. (a) Blood pressure 140/90 mm Hg or higher; (b) temperature 38° C (100.4° F) or higher
11. Use soft, indirect lighting. Keep the temperature comfortable with a fan or damp, cool washcloths. Have the woman wear socks for cold feet. Keep the woman reasonably clean by changing her underpad as often as needed. Offer ice chips or a wet washcloth to wet her lips. Remind her to empty her bladder at least every 2 hours. Encourage her to change positions frequently, assuming the position of comfort (except the supine position). Offer a shower, whirlpool, or other water therapy.

Labeling

1. Refer to Procedure 13-1 on p. 274-275 to complete this exercise. Problem a: The nurse would feel a firm but irregular mass that moves with the fetal trunk in the fundus; a smooth, convex surface would be felt on the mother's right, and multiple nodular masses ("small parts") would be felt on her left side rather than her right; a hard, rounded mass would be felt in the suprapubic area, and the nurse would not be able to displace it upward; the cephalic prominence (the fetal forehead in this case) would be felt on the mother's left side. Problem b: The nurse would feel a hard, round mass in the fundus that could be moved without moving the fetal trunk; a smooth, convex surface would be felt on the far left side of the uterus, and nodular masses would be felt on the right side; a softer mass would be felt in her suprapubic area, and it could be easily displaced upward; the fourth maneuver is omitted if the fetus is in a breech presentation.
Illustration shows the fetus in a left occiput anterior (LOA) position rather than ROA as stated in labeling problem a. Problem b is a reversal of locations for head and buttocks, with the fetal head being in the fundus and fetal buttocks presenting at the cervix.

Check Yourself

1, b; 2, d; 3, a; 4, c; 5, d; 6, b; 7, d; 8, a; 9, b; 10, d

Case Study

1. Regular contractions that have increased in duration, intensity, and frequency suggest true labor. Irregular contractions and those that do not intensify suggest false labor. In addition, discomfort is usually felt in her back or sweeping around to her lower abdomen. Erin should be instructed to come to the birth center if she thinks her membranes may have ruptured, even if she is not having contractions.
2. Priorities are to (a) assess the FHR and, if membranes have ruptured, the color, odor, and character of the amniotic fluid; (b) assess Erin's vital signs; and (c) determine the nearness to birth by evaluating contractions and cervical dilation.
3. Either a pH or fern test or both are the two tests that are often used to evaluate whether the membranes have ruptured.
4. Active phase of first-stage labor
5. The FHR is normal for a term fetus, and it is reassuring that the FHR accelerates.
6. Except for the greenish color, the amniotic fluid is normal. The amniotic fluid is green because the fetus passed meconium before birth. Fetal problems may or may not exist.
7. Cephalic; right occiput posterior (ROP)

8. Assuming any of several upright positions and leaning forward during contractions; hands and knees; firm sacral pressure

9. Delayed pushing may be encouraged until Erin has a more intense urge to push. When Erin pushes, she should avoid prolonged breath-holding. She can be taught to take a deep breath and exhale it and then take another deep breath and push for 4 to 6 seconds at a time while exhaling. A final deep breath at the end of the contraction helps her relax.

10. The exact time to position Erin for birth will depend on how fast she has labored thus far. In general, a woman having her first baby is positioned for the birth when the fetal head crowns and remains visible between contractions.

11. The 1-minute Apgar score will be 9, with one point deducted for the baby's bluish hands and feet.

12. (a) Suction to remove excess secretions as needed; position infant flat or on one side with the head flat or slightly elevated. (b) Dry the baby quickly, including the head; place in a prewarmed radiant warmer or in skin-to-skin contact with a parent, which can be used to position the baby's head favorably; use a cap on the baby's dry head to reduce heat loss from that area when not in the radiant warmer.

13. The first 1 to 4 hours after the placenta delivers is the fourth stage of labor.

14. Firmness, height, and position of the uterine fundus; vital signs; amount of lochia; and observing and intervening for a full bladder help prevent hemorrhage caused by the bladder's interference with uterine contraction.

15. Cold packs to the perineal area; analgesics; a warm blanket to limit the common postbirth chill

Intrapartum Fetal Surveillance

Learning Activities

1. Match each term with its definition (a-g).

_____ Amnioinfusion

_____ Baseline fetal heart rate

_____ Nuchal cord

_____ Periodic fetal heart rate changes

_____ Tocolytic

_____ Uterine resting tone

_____ Variability

a. Fluctuations in the baseline fetal heart rate

b. Cord around the fetus's neck

c. Fetal heart rate when the uterus is at rest

d. Temporary, recurrent changes in the fetal heart rate

e. Infusion of a sterile solution into the amniotic cavity to reduce cord compression

f. Muscle tension when the uterus is not contracting

g. Drug that reduces uterine muscle contractions

2. List the five factors that affect fetal oxygenation.

a.

b.

c.

d.

e.

3. Explain how each of the following fetal factors influences the fetal heart rate.

a. Autonomic nervous system

b. Baroreceptors

c. Chemoreceptors

d. Adrenal glands

e. Central nervous system

4. Explain how each of the following factors can reduce fetal oxygenation. How would you explain each in simple terms to a laboring woman?

a. Maternal hypotension

b. Maternal hypertension

c. Maternal hypoxia

d. Hypertonic uterine activity

e. Placental disruptions

f. Umbilical cord blood flow compression

g. Fetal bradycardia or tachycardia

5. List the advantages and limitations of the two methods of intrapartum fetal assessment—auscultation with palpation of contractions and electronic fetal monitoring.

	Auscultation with Palpation	*Electronic Fetal Monitoring*
Advantages		
Limitations		

6. What must the nurse consider when evaluating intrauterine pressures from a solid catheter versus a fluid-filled catheter?

7. Define these terms that describe the fetal heart rate.
   a. Normal

   b. Bradycardia

   c. Tachycardia

8. List factors that may decrease variability.

9. Why is variability an important component of fetal heart pattern evaluation? Under what circumstances might variability normally be minimal? Why?

10. Describe each fetal heart rate periodic change, list possible causes, note whether the change is reassuring or not, and give the basic actions to take if nonreassuring.

Periodic Change	Appearance on Strip	Possible Causes	Reassuring or Nonreassuring (with Nursing Actions)
Accelerations			
Early decelerations			
Late decelerations			
Variable decelerations			

11. Describe three methods that can be used during labor to clarify the fetal condition.

a.

b.

c.

12. List possible nursing or medical interventions to identify or correct the cause of a nonreassuring fetal monitor pattern.

    a. Identifying the cause

    b. Increasing placental perfusion

    c. Increasing maternal oxygen saturation

    d. Reducing umbilical cord compression

13. Describe the primary purpose of amnioinfusion. Describe how it is done and basic nursing care involved.

Labeling

1. Label the following on the monitor strip, assuming a paper speed of 3 cm/min.
  a. 1-minute interval
  b. 10-second interval
  c. Fetal heart rate grid
  d. Uterine activity grid
  e. Normal range of fetal heart rate at term

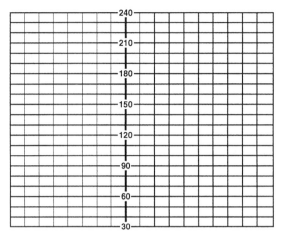

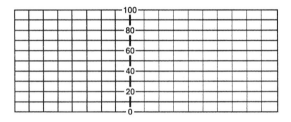

Check Yourself

1. Firm contractions that occur every 2 to 2½ minutes and last 100 seconds (1 minute, 40 seconds) may reduce fetal oxygen supply because they
  a. Cause fetal bradycardia and reduce oxygen concentration
  b. Activate the fetal sympathetic nervous system
  c. Reduce time for oxygen exchange in the placenta
  d. Suppress the normal variability of the fetal heart

2. The expected response of the fetal heart rate of a term fetus to movement is
  a. Suppression of normal variability for at least 15 seconds
  b. Acceleration of 15 or more beats per minute (bpm) for 15 seconds
  c. Increase in variability by 15 bpm for 10 minutes
  d. Acceleration followed by deceleration of the heart rate

3. The nurse notes a pattern of variable decelerations to 75 bpm on the fetal monitor. The initial nursing action should be to
  a. Reposition the woman
  b. Administer oxygen
  c. Increase the intravenous (IV) infusion
  d. Stimulate the fetal scalp

4. The woman who uses cocaine is more likely to have which pattern on the electronic fetal heart monitor?
  a. Intermittent tachycardia
  b. Periodic accelerations
  c. Variable decelerations
  d. Late decelerations

5. The tocotransducer should be placed
   a. In the suprapubic area
   b. In the fundal area
   c. Over the xiphoid process
   d. Within the uterus

6. The nurse should respond to incomplete uterine relaxation between contractions by
   a. Increasing the rate of IV fluid
   b. Having the woman push with contractions
   c. Contacting the physician for a tocolytic order
   d. Initiating an amnioinfusion with Ringer's lactate

7. A woman is admitted in possible labor at 34 weeks of gestation. She is monitored with the external fetal monitor while on her left side. The nurse should periodically assess the contractions by palpation, primarily because
   a. It makes the woman feel more like her pregnancy is normal.
   b. Palpation identifies whether the fetus has changed its presentation.
   c. Contractions may not be sensed by the tocotransducer while she is on her side.
   d. The tocotransducer is not accurate for actual intensity and uterine resting tone.

8. Choose the important precaution to be taken when a solid intrauterine pressure catheter is used to monitor uterine contractions during labor.
   a. The pressure reflects the pressure of the fluid above, as well as the pressure of the contraction.
   b. The fluid that fills the catheter must be warmed to room temperature.
   c. Understand that pressures within the fluid-filled catheter are higher than those in the solid catheter.
   d. Fluid-filled catheters cannot be used when a spiral electrode is applied.

9. The nurse notes a pattern of decelerations on the fetal monitor that begins shortly after the contraction begins and returns to baseline just before the contraction is over. The correct nursing response is to
   a. Give the woman oxygen by face mask at 8 to 10 L/min
   b. Position the woman on her opposite side
   c. Increase the rate of the woman's IV fluid
   d. Continue to observe and record the normal pattern

Developing Insight

1. Look at fetal monitor strips in your clinical facility. Identify the following about each.
   a. Baseline rate
   b. Presence of variability
   c. Periodic changes
   d. Contraction frequency, duration, and intensity
   e. Nursing interventions for nonreassuring patterns
   f. Fetal responses to nursing interventions

2. Your friend is 7 months pregnant and is uncertain about whether she wants to have electronic fetal monitoring. Develop a plan to explain the pros and cons of each method of fetal surveillance during labor.

3. Analyze each of the following strips as indicated. Determine basic nursing for each. An external uterine activity monitor is being used in strip a. Strips b and c use an intrauterine pressure catheter to record uterine activity.

a.

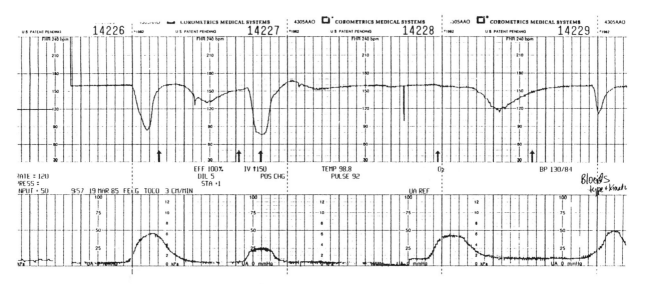

Baseline fetal heart rate (FHR) is _____ bpm.

FHR variability is _____ bpm.

Are there any periodic patterns? Which?

Contraction frequency is every _____ minutes.

Contraction duration is _____ seconds.

What nursing actions are appropriate? What is the rationale for each?

b.

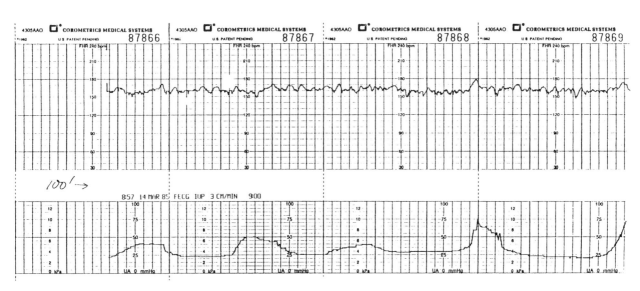

Baseline FHR is _____ bpm.

FHR variability is _____ bpm.

Are there any periodic patterns? Which?

Contraction frequency is every _____ minutes.

Contraction duration is _____ seconds.

Contraction intensity is _____ mm Hg.

Uterine resting tone is _____ mm Hg.

What nursing actions are appropriate? What is the rationale for each?

c.

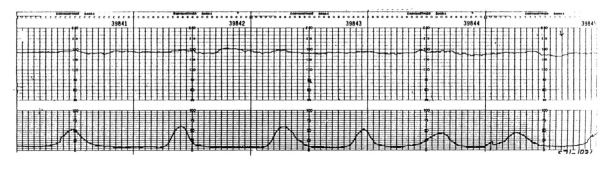

Baseline FHR is _____ bpm.

FHR variability is _____ bpm.

Are there any periodic patterns? Which?

Contraction frequency is every _____ minutes.

Contraction duration is _____ seconds.

Contraction intensity is _____ mm Hg.

Uterine resting tone is _____ mm Hg.

What nursing actions are appropriate? What is the rationale for each?

ANSWERS TO SELECTED QUESTIONS

Learning Activities

1. e, c, b, d, g, f, a
2. (In any order) (a) Adequate maternal blood volume and flow to the placenta. (b) Adequate oxygen saturation in the maternal blood. (c) Adequate exchange of oxygen and carbon dioxide in the placenta. (d) Open circulatory path between the placenta and fetus through umbilical cord vessels. (e) Normal fetal circulatory and oxygen-carrying functions.
3. (a) Sympathetic stimulation increases the heart rate and strengthens the heart contractions to increase cardiac output by releasing epinephrine and norepinephrine. (b) Baroreceptors sense blood pressure increases in the carotid arch and major arteries to slow the heart and reduce the blood pressure, thus reducing cardiac output. (c) Chemoreceptors in the medulla oblongata, aortic arch, and carotid bodies sense changes in oxygen, carbon dioxide, and pH to increase the heart rate if hypoxia, hypercapnia, and acidosis, respectively, are not prolonged. (d) Adrenal glands secrete epinephrine and norepinephrine in response to stress and release aldosterone to cause retention of sodium and water, thus increasing the blood volume. (e) The fetal cerebral cortex causes the fetal heart rate (FHR) to increase during fetal movement and decrease during fetal sleep; the hypothalamus coordinates the branches of the autonomic nervous system. The medulla oblongata maintains balance between forces that speed and slow the FHR.
4. Refer to text, pp. 303-304, to complete this exercise.
5. Refer to text, pp. 304-305 and 307, to complete this exercise.
6. The pressures from a solid intrauterine pressure catheter are slightly higher than those of the fluid-filled catheter. The fluid-filled catheter is sensitive to the height of the catheter tip in relation to the transducer.
7. If the fetus is at term: (a) Lower limit of 110 and upper limit of 160 beats per minute (bpm). (b) Rate less than 110 bpm that persists for at least 10 minutes. Rate of 100 to 110 may be normal in the term fetus. (c) Rate greater than 160 bpm that persists for at least 10 minutes.
8. Maternal: narcotics or other sedatives; recent alcohol or drug ingestion; acidemia or hypoxemia. Fetal: tachycardia; prematurity; decreased central nervous system oxygenation; abnormalities of the central nervous system or heart; anomalies that may affect FHR; fetal sleep.
9. Variability reflects normal function of the autonomic nervous system, which helps the fetus adapt to the stress of labor. Minimal variability might be normal in prematurity or fetal sleep or after maternal narcotic or sedative administration, because these conditions do not reflect reduced nervous system oxygenation. Fetal sleep would be temporary, and variability should reappear when the fetus awakens, usually in approximately 40 minutes at term. Narcotic effects would last longer but would still be temporary.
10. Refer to text, pp. 313-320, and Table 14-1, p. 318 to complete this exercise.
11. (In any order) (a) Fetal scalp stimulation; (b) vibroacoustic stimulation; (c) fetal scalp blood sampling
12. (a) Check blood pressure to identify hypotension or hypertension, contractions to identify uterine hyperactivity, and recent maternal medications to identify sedative effects; perform vaginal examination to identify prolapsed cord; initiate internal monitoring to provide more accuracy. (b) Change position to reduce aortocaval compression; discontinue oxytocin or administer tocolytics to reduce uterine activity; increase nonadditive intravenous (IV) fluid to correct hypovolemia or vasodilation. (c) Administer 100% oxygen at 8 to 10 L/min through a snug face mask. (d) Reposition or perform amnioinfusion to reduce umbilical cord compression.
13. Add fluid to create a cushion around the umbilical cord. Use to dilute thick meconium in amniotic fluid has not been found beneficial. Warm and sterile isotonic fluid is infused into the uterine cavity. Nursing care is to keep the woman dry as fluid leaks continuously from her vagina. Overdistention of the uterus may be relieved by releasing some of the fluid.

Labeling

Refer to Figure 14-4 on p. 308.

Check Yourself

1, c; 2, b; 3, a; 4, d; 5, b; 6, c; 7, d; 8, a; 9, d

Developing Insight

3. a. FHR baseline is approximately 160 bpm; variability is 0 bpm (absent). The first, second, and fourth decelerations are variable, and the third is a late deceleration. Contraction frequency is every 2 to 4 minutes, with duration of 40 to 50 seconds. Nursing interventions include repositioning to reduce cord compression, discontinuing oxytocin if infusing, increasing the rate of a nonadditive IV fluid, and giving oxygen by face mask. The birth attendant should be notified promptly.

b. FHR baseline is 150 to 170 bpm, with variability averaging 15 to 20 bpm. There are no periodic changes. Contractions are approximately every 2 to 2½ minutes, with duration of 40 to 60 seconds. Contraction intensity in this 10-minute strip ranges from 40 to 75 mm Hg and the uterine resting tone is high at 25 mm Hg. Nursing actions include checking the fluid-filled catheter for factors that might artificially raise the uterine resting tone. If uterine resting tone is truly elevated, measures to identify and correct its cause (e.g., possible placental abruption) should be taken. The birth attendant should be notified.

c. FHR baseline averages 170 bpm, with almost no variability. Late decelerations are seen with the first, second, fifth, and sixth contractions. Contractions are every 2 to 4 minutes, duration is approximately 40 to 50 seconds, and uterine resting tone is 10 to 15 mm Hg. Intensity averages 40 to 60 mm Hg. Nursing actions are to evaluate the gestation to identify prematurity as a factor in reduced variability, to recognize that reduced or absent variability occurs with tachycardia, and to assess the mother for signs of infection (elevated temperature and pulse, foul-smelling amniotic fluid). Maternal blood pressure identifies hypotension or hypertension that could contribute to reduced placental blood flow. The woman should be positioned to avoid aortocaval compression.

Pain Management during Childbirth

Learning Activities

1. Match each term with its definition (a-j).

_____ Agonist

_____ Analgesia

_____ Anesthesia

_____ Antagonist

_____ Cleansing breath

_____ Endorphin

_____ Habituation

_____ Paced breathing

_____ Sellick maneuver

_____ Valsalva maneuver

a. Blocking effect of a drug

b. Holding the breath while pushing against a closed glottis

c. Reduced effectiveness of a pain management method after prolonged use

d. Loss of sensation with or without loss of consciousness

e. Blocking the esophagus by pressing the trachea against it

f. A deep breath taken at the beginning and end of each contraction

g. Relief of pain without loss of consciousness

h. Causing a physiologic effect

i. Natural substance similar to morphine

j. Learned breathing techniques used during labor

2. Explain the difference between pain threshold and pain tolerance. What factors can influence a woman's pain tolerance during labor, either positively or negatively?

3. How can excessive maternal pain reduce fetal oxygenation?

4. How is labor affected when the fetus is in an occiput posterior (OP) position?

5. Describe key features of each type of breathing technique and variations of each type that the woman may choose.
   a. Cleansing breath

   b. Slow-paced breathing

   c. Modified-paced breathing

   d. Patterned-paced breathing

6. What breathing technique can help the woman avoid pushing too early?

7. Describe hyperventilation and nursing interventions to help a woman correct the problem.

8. Compare and contrast open-glottis pushing with closed-glottis pushing.

9. What is the purpose of giving a test dose before performing an epidural block? What would be signs of problems after the test dose, and what causes these signs?

10. What causes the following adverse reactions to epidural block analgesia or anesthesia? What can be done to prevent or correct each?
   a. Hypotension

   b. Bladder distention

   c. Prolonged second stage

   d. Catheter migration

   e. Fever

11. In which regional anesthesia method is it desirable to obtain cerebrospinal fluid (CSF)? Why?

12. Under what two circumstances should butorphanol (Stadol) or nalbuphine (Nubain) be avoided when a laboring woman is being medicated?

13. If an infant receives naloxone (Narcan), why should the nurse continue to monitor the infant for respiratory depression?

14. Complete the following table on intrapartum pain-relief methods.

Technique	Advantages	Disadvantages	Adverse Effects	Nursing Care
Systemic analgesics				
Epidural block				
Intrathecal opioids				
Subarachnoid block				
Local infiltration				
Pudendal block				
General anesthesia				

15. List methods to relieve pain of a spinal headache.

Check Yourself

1. Firm sacral pressure is likely to be most helpful in which situation?
   a. Rapid labor and birth
   b. Fetal occiput posterior position
   c. Oxytocin induction of labor
   d. If analgesics should be avoided

2. During active labor, a woman complains of tingly, stiff fingers when using patterned-paced breathing. In response, the nurse should focus primarily on helping her
   a. Slow her respiratory rate
   b. Maintain a focal point
   c. Relax her upper extremities
   d. Push with an open glottis

3. When one is stocking a cart for epidural analgesia, the most important nursing action is to
   a. Add several 50-ml bags of intravenous (IV) saline
   b. Place anticoagulant drugs to allow rapid access
   c. Verify that no epidural drugs have preservatives
   d. Provide an indwelling catheterization tray

4. A resident physician orders meperidine (Demerol), 35 mg, and hydroxyzine (Vistaril), 25 mg, by slow IV push for a laboring woman. The appropriate nursing action is to
   a. Remind the physician that hydroxyzine is not given by IV push
   b. Give the meperidine by IV push and the hydroxyzine by deep intramuscular (IM) administration
   c. Dilute the two drugs before giving them by slow IV push
   d. Give the drugs as ordered by the physician

5. The appropriate nursing action for a woman who has a postspinal headache is to
   a. Keep her bed in a semi-Fowler's position
   b. Encourage intake of fluids that she enjoys
   c. Have her ambulate at least every 4 hours
   d. Restrict intake of high-carbohydrate foods

6. A woman having her first baby is trying to use breathing techniques during labor but has difficulty concentrating. She is dilated 3 cm, she is 80% effaced, and the station is 0. What nursing measure can best help her?
   a. Encourage her to change to a different breathing pattern.
   b. Have a family member other than her husband coach her.
   c. Give her a very small dose of narcotic that is ordered as needed (prn).
   d. Help her find a specific point in the room to focus on.

7. A woman must have general anesthesia for planned cesarean birth because of previous back surgery. The nurse should therefore expect to administer
   a. Naltrexone (Trexan)
   b. An oral barbiturate
   c. Ranitidine (Zantac)
   d. Promethazine (Phenergan)

Developing Insight

1. Make a plan to help a woman with the anxiety and fear that can accompany labor. Use the experience of a woman you have helped care for, that of a friend or relative, or your own experience when making your plan.

2. You may need to help a woman correct her labor breathing or breathe with her while she is in labor, so you must know breathing techniques well. Practice each technique until you are comfortable with it, and then teach the techniques to a family member.

3. Try the breathing techniques in a stressful situation. For example, take a cleansing breath when you begin your next nursing test. Breathe slowly and deliberately as you take the test. Did it help reduce your stress?

4. Talk to an anesthesia clinician in your clinical facility about how he or she compensates for the normal changes of pregnancy when giving anesthesia.

Case Study

Alice is a 16-year-old primigravida in the latent phase of first-stage labor. She did not attend prepared childbirth classes. She is very anxious and tense, crying during each contraction. Her cervix is dilated to 3 cm, station −1, effacement 90%, and the membranes are ruptured (amniotic fluid is clear). Her baseline vital signs are pulse, 92 beats per minute (bpm); respirations, 24 breaths per minute; and blood pressure, 120/70 mm Hg. Fetal heart rate (FHR) is 126 to 136 bpm with average variability. Her 17-year-old husband is at her side but seems very frustrated and helpless. Her parents live out of town; her husband's parents are with the couple.

1. What assumptions must the nurse be careful to avoid when caring for Alice?

2. What initial nursing interventions are appropriate to help Alice cope with her contractions?

3. Can Alice be taught breathing techniques at this time? If so, how should the nurse approach the teaching?

4. Are analgesics desirable for Alice at this time? Why or why not?

Alice progresses to 6-cm cervical dilation, effacement 100%, and fetal station 0. Maternal and fetal vital signs remain stable. Alice wants "something stronger" for the pain.

5. What pharmacologic options are possible for Alice, based on the information given?

Alice receives epidural block analgesia.

6. What nursing care is essential related to the block? Why?

Alice gives birth to a 2380-g (6-lb, 2-oz) girl. Apgar scores are 7 at 1 minute and 9 at 5 minutes.

7. What are appropriate nursing measures related to Alice's epidural while she is in the recovery area?

ANSWERS TO SELECTED QUESTIONS

Learning Activities

1. h, g, d, a, f, i, c, j, e, b
2. Pain threshold is the minimum stimulus that a person perceives as painful; it is relatively constant under different conditions. Pain tolerance is the maximum amount of pain a person is willing to endure; it may change with the circumstances. Factors influencing pain tolerance during labor include intensity of labor, readiness of the cervix to dilate with the force of contractions, fetal position, pelvic size and shape, maternal fatigue and hunger, or interventions of caregivers (either a positive or negative influence).
3. Excess maternal pain can result in fear and anxiety, which stimulate the mother's sympathetic nervous system to release substances that simultaneously cause vasoconstriction and pooling of blood in the mother's vascular system, plus a higher uterine muscle tone with reduction of effective contractions. The net effect is that blood flow to and from the placenta falls and labor contractions are less effective, thus prolonging labor.
4. The fetal occiput is pushed against the woman's sacral promontory with each contraction, causing intense back pain. In addition, the fetus must usually rotate into the occiput anterior position to be born, so labor is often longer.
5. (a) The cleansing breath releases tension, provides oxygen, clears the mind to focus on relaxing, signals labor partner of contraction's beginning or end; may be taken in any way comfortable. (b) Slow-paced breathing enhances relaxation and allows the woman to concentrate on relaxation rather than number of breaths; she may use nose, mouth, or combination breathing. (c) Modified-paced breathing uses shallow, but rapid, breathing, and it may be combined with slow-paced breathing. (d) Focus on pattern of breathing interferes with pain impulse transmission; some may make special sound ("hee" and "hoo"); the woman may vary number of breaths before blowing.
6. Blowing prevents glottis closure and breath-holding.
7. Rapid, deep breathing results in loss of carbon dioxide, eventually resulting in respiratory alkalosis. Woman feels dizzy or lightheaded, with numbness and tingling of fingers and lips; tetany, stiffness of the face and lips, or carpopedal spasm may occur. Breathing into a paper bag or cupped hands causes rebreathing of carbon dioxide and correction of alkalosis.
8. Traditional closed-glottis pushing may result in impaired blood flow to uterus, is fatiguing for the woman, and has not proven to significantly shorten second stage. Open-glottis pushing improves maternal-fetal oxygenation and is more physiologic, but the second stage may be longer.
9. The test dose is given to identify inadvertent dural or intravascular puncture before injection of the full dose of the anesthetic drug. Evidence of these problems includes rapid and intense motor and sensory block (subdural or subarachnoid injection) or numbness of the tongue and lips, lightheadedness, dizziness, and tinnitus (intravascular injection).
10. Refer to text p. 342-343 to answer the question about causes for each adverse reaction. To prevent or correct each cause, the nurse or birth attendant must: (a) Prehydrate the woman with a minimum of 500 to 1000 mL of intravenous (IV) solution. Ephedrine in 5- to 10-mg increments may be needed. (b) Check the bladder for distention, and catheterize as needed. (c) Coach the woman to push if she does not have an urge to push. (d) Observe for excess anesthesia, one-sided block, a too-high block, or loss of anesthesia after its initiation. Report if he or she questions the intactness of the epidural. (e) Observe the maternal temperature every 2 hours after membranes rupture and report a temperature of 38° C (100.4° F) or higher. Although slight temperature elevations are common with epidurals, observe for signs of infection, such as foul- or strong-smelling amniotic fluid or fluid that is cloudy or yellow.
11. The subarachnoid block (SAB) punctures the dura and arachnoid membranes, entering the space that contains cerebrospinal fluid (CSF). Appearance of a few drops of CSF confirms the correct location for injection of the anesthetic drug for this block.
12. These drugs have combined opioid agonist-antagonist effects and should not be given to a woman who has had a recent dose of a pure opioid agonist (may reverse effectiveness of first drug) or to a woman who is addicted to opiates such as heroin (may precipitate acute withdrawal). These drugs also have a ceiling effect and are unlikely to provide sufficient analgesia for the entire labor.
13. The duration of action for naloxone is shorter than for most of the opioids it reverses. Respiratory depression could recur until effects of the opioid drug have abated.
14. Consult text, pp. 341-355, and Table 15-2, pp. 354-355, to complete this exercise.
15. Bed rest with oral or IV hydration; blood patch

Check Yourself

1, b; 2, a; 3, c; 4, a; 5, b; 6, d; 7, c

Case Study

1. The nurse must be careful to avoid assumptions such as that the pregnancy was unplanned, that Alice did not have prenatal care, and that she and her husband cannot learn nonpharmacologic pain management methods or that she would want an epidural right away. Think of other assumptions that nurses should avoid. Consider assumptions nurses might have about teen parents being married.

2. Initial interventions are to tell Alice and her husband that her labor pattern is normal right now and show them data that indicate that mother and fetus are doing well. The nurse should speak calmly and in a soothing voice, conveying to Alice and her husband that they can have confidence in their caregivers and that Alice is capable of giving birth.

3. The nurse should teach Alice simple breathing and relaxation techniques between contractions. Say something such as, "I'm going to teach you how to breathe so that you can cope with labor better," in a positive manner that conveys the expectation that the techniques will work, rather than doing the teaching in a tentative manner. Give liberal positive feedback when Alice uses the techniques taught, and give her husband positive feedback for his coaching.

4. It would be better for Alice to delay taking medication until labor is in the active phase. Administration of analgesics or epidural block analgesia too early can slow labor progress. However, this fact must be balanced against the adverse effects of excessive pain and anxiety and the woman's need for pharmacologic pain relief.

5. At this point, Alice could probably receive either an opioid analgesic or an epidural block.

6. The nurse must prehydrate Alice with a minimum of 500 to 1000 mL of IV solution, check her blood pressure frequently to detect hypotension, and observe the fetal heart rate (FHR) for signs of reduced placental perfusion that can occur with maternal hypotension. The nurse must also observe for bladder distention related to loss of sensation and high volumes of IV fluids. Alice may need coaching to push during the second stage if she cannot feel the urge. In addition, the nurse must be alert for signs of catheter migration or maternal fever or infection. The nurse should explain every intervention and its rationale simply.

7. The nurse must continue to observe for bladder distention during both first- and second-stage labor, which can result in poor uterine contraction and postpartum hemorrhage. Return of sensation must be documented. The nurse must assist Alice to the bathroom at first in case she still has reduced sensation or hypotension that could result in a fall. If catheterization is needed any time during labor, the nurse should first explain the reasons and procedures simply.

Nursing Care during Obstetric Procedures

Learning Activities

1. Match each term with its definition (a-h).

_____ Augmentation

_____ Chignon

_____ Dystocia

_____ Iatrogenic

_____ Montevideo unit

_____ Nuchal cord

_____ Pfannenstiel

_____ Piper

a. Newborn scalp edema caused by a vacuum extractor

b. "Bikini" skin incision

c. Forceps used to assist vaginal breech birth

d. Method to calculate the intensity of uterine contractions over 10 minutes

e. Difficult or prolonged labor

f. Adverse condition resulting from treatment

g. Cord around the fetal neck

h. Stimulation to improve effectiveness of spontaneous labor contractions

2. List the potential complications of amniotomy.

3. Complete the following table about nursing assessments after amniotomy.

Assessment	Expected Findings	Abnormal Findings
Fetal heart rate (FHR)		
Amniotic fluid character		

4. List three nursing measures after use of prostaglandin E$_2$ to ripen the cervix and the rationale for each.
   a.

   b.

   c.

5. Describe fetal and maternal nursing assessments associated with oxytocin infusion. What are signs of problems?
   a. Fetal assessments

   b. Maternal assessments

6. List nursing interventions if fetal or maternal assessments are not reassuring when oxytocin induction or augmentation of labor is being performed.

7. Explain the purpose of each aspect of care for the woman having external version.
   a. Nonstress test or biophysical profile

   b. Epidural block or sedative

   c. Ultrasound

   d. Tocolytic drug

   e. Rh immune globulin

   f. Fetal heart rate monitoring

   g. Uterine activity monitoring

8. Describe nursing care associated with a forceps- or vacuum extractor–assisted birth. What is the rationale for each? Are there contraindications for either method?
   a. Maternal

   b. Fetal/neonatal

   c. Contraindications

9. Write a simply worded explanation that you might give to a woman immediately after birth about why you are placing a cold pack on her perineal area. How would you explain the change to warm packs the next day?

10. A woman gave birth to her first baby, a boy weighing 4086 g (9 lb). Low forceps with a mediolateral episiotomy were required. List three nursing diagnoses or collaborative problems that would be expected during the first 12 hours after birth and appropriate nursing measures for each.

Nursing Diagnosis or Collaborative Problem	Nursing Interventions

11. Explain why cesarean birth is not always easy for the newborn.

12. Explain the rationale for each intervention associated with cesarean birth.
    a. Maintaining NPO (nothing by mouth) status

    b. Placing a wedge under one hip

    c. Complete blood count, coagulation studies, blood type and crossmatch

    d. Intravenous (IV) antibiotic

    e. Indwelling catheter

Labeling

1. Draw a median (midline) and a mediolateral episiotomy on the following figures. List advantages and disadvantages of each.

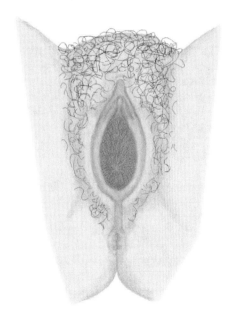 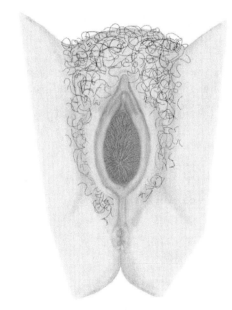

	Median (Midline) Episiotomy	*Mediolateral Episiotomy*
Advantages		
Disadvantages		

2. Draw a vertical and a Pfannenstiel skin incision for cesarean birth on the following drawing. List advantages and disadvantages of each.

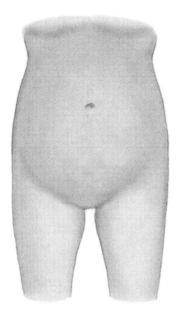
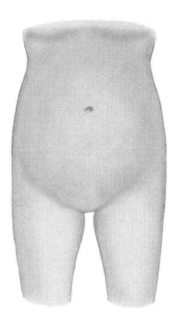

	Vertical Skin Incision	*Pfannenstiel Skin Incision*
Advantages		
Disadvantages		

3. Draw a low transverse, low vertical, and classic uterine incision for cesarean birth on the following drawing. List advantages and disadvantages of each. Rank them in the order of preference, explaining why each has that rank.

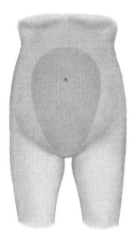 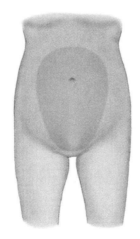 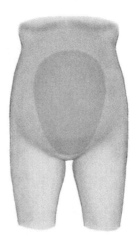

	Low Transverse Uterine Incision	*Low Vertical Uterine Incision*	*Classic Uterine Incision*
Advantages			
Disadvantages			
Preference rank and why			

Check Yourself

1. After the physician performs an amniotomy, the fluid is dark green with a mild odor and the FHR is 130 to 140 beats per minute (bpm). The most appropriate nursing care is to
a. Take the woman's temperature hourly until delivery
b. Monitor the fetus more closely for nonreassuring signs
c. Tell the woman that she cannot have anything by mouth
d. Observe the woman closely for hypotension

2. Choose the correct setup for oxytocin induction of labor.
   a. Oxytocin is mixed with an electrolyte solution and delivered as a single infusion.
   b. Oxytocin is mixed with normal saline to equal 10 mL and given by slow IV push.
   c. Oxytocin is begun at a rapid rate; its rate is decreased as labor progresses.
   d. Oxytocin is given as a secondary infusion and is controlled by an infusion pump.

3. A method to prepare the cervix for induction of labor is
   a. Prostaglandin vaginal inserts
   b. Fetal fibronectin
   c. Oral oxytocin tablets
   d. Amniotomy

4. Choose the nursing assessment that is most likely to occur with hypertonic uterine contractions.
   a. Foul-smelling amniotic fluid
   b. Contraction interval of 90 seconds
   c. FHR of 80 to 100 bpm
   d. Maternal pulse of 80 to 90 bpm

5. A woman has a successful external version to change her fetal position from breech to cephalic at 38 weeks of gestation. Choose the postprocedure nursing observation that would indicate she should not be released to go home.
   a. FHR is 135 to 145 bpm with average variability.
   b. Occasional mild, brief contractions occur.
   c. Maternal temperature is 37.3° C (99.2° F), and pulse is 90 bpm.
   d. Vaginal discharge is a pale and watery fluid.

6. Parents of an infant born with a forceps-assisted vaginal birth ask about small reddened areas on the infant's cheeks. The nurse should tell them that the areas
   a. Are temporary and will disappear
   b. Are typical of all vaginal births
   c. Will be reported to the physician
   d. May lead to a serious infection

7. A urinary catheter should be readily available when a woman with no indwelling catheter has a forceps-assisted birth because
   a. Emergency cesarean birth may be required
   b. Edema reduces the woman's sensation to void after birth
   c. A full bladder reduces available room in the pelvis
   d. A large median or mediolateral episiotomy is likely

8. During the recovery period after low vacuum extraction birth with a median episiotomy, the nurse should
   a. Assess for purulent drainage from the episiotomy
   b. Apply cold packs to the perineal area promptly
   c. Expect a larger quantity of lochia rubra drainage
   d. Limit oral intake to ice chips until transfer to a room

9. Choose correct preoperative teaching before planned cesarean birth.
   a. Oral intake will be limited to clear fluids for 12 hours before surgery.
   b. IV fluids are usually continued for 2 days after birth.
   c. The woman will be asked to take deep breaths and cough regularly after birth.
   d. The nurse will help her ambulate to the restroom to urinate 4 hours after birth.

10. The best method to prevent hemorrhage after cesarean birth is to
   a. Provide regular analgesia to enhance urination
   b. Reposition the woman from side to side
   c. Observe vital signs for falling blood pressure
   d. Assess the uterine fundus regularly for firmness

Developing Insight

1. Observe a cesarean birth, and compare the sequence of events with those of vaginal birth. What are the similarities and differences?

2. What measures do you see the nursing staff taking to keep the emphasis on the birth experience rather than on surgery when a woman has cesarean birth?

3. Which is more common in your clinical facility? What is the source of your data for each answer?
   a. Forceps- or vacuum extraction–assisted birth

   b. Forceps or vacuum extraction births or cesarean births

Case Study

Linda is a gravida 3, para 2, at 41 weeks of gestation. She is scheduled for oxytocin induction of labor. Her first two pregnancies ended at 39 and 40 weeks, and the babies weighed 3996 g (8 lb, 13 oz) and 4394 g (9 lb, 11 oz).

1. What is the probable reason for Linda's induction?

2. What tests might be performed before her induction?

Linda's initial assessments are normal, and the FHR is reassuring. She is having an occasional light contraction but no regular contractions.

3. How should the nurse set up the oxytocin infusion? What is the rationale for setting up the infusion in this manner?

After 3 hours, Linda's cervix is dilated to 3 cm, effacement is 80%, and the fetal station is −1. Contractions are every 4 to 5 minutes, last 45 seconds, and are of moderate intensity. The FHR is 132 to 148 bpm. The physician decides to perform an amniotomy.

4. What nursing measures are appropriate before and after the amniotomy?

5. Should there be any change in the oxytocin infusion at this time? Why or why not?

Linda's labor progresses, and she is having contractions approximately every 2 to 3 minutes, of 90 to 100 seconds' duration, and firm. FHR baseline on the monitor averages 130 to 140 bpm with occasional accelerations to the 150- to 160-bpm range. She is dilated to 7 cm, effacement is 90%, and the fetal station is −1.

6. Should there be any change in her oxytocin infusion at this time? Why or why not?

Despite adequate contractions, Linda's cervical dilation does not progress beyond 7 cm and she will have a cesarean birth.

7. What nursing measures are appropriate for the planned birth?

Linda delivers a 4624-g (10-lb, 3-oz) girl by low transverse cesarean birth.

8. What nursing care is appropriate for Linda while in the recovery phase?

ANSWERS TO SELECTED QUESTIONS

Learning Activities

1. h, a, e, f, d, g, b, c
2. Prolapse of the umbilical cord, infection, and placental abruption
3. Refer to p. 362 to complete this exercise.
4. (In any order) (a) Have the woman lie flat for 15 to 20 minutes to reduce leakage. (b) Observe the fetal heart rate (FHR) for changes that may occur with uterine contractions. (c) Assess for excessive contractions that can reduce fetal oxygen supply (see also Chapters 12 and 14).
5. (a) Assess the FHR every 15 minutes during first-stage labor and every 5 minutes during second-stage labor. Problems may be indicated by tachycardia (>160 beats per minute [bpm]), bradycardia (<110 bpm), late decelerations, and reduced FHR variability. (b) Assess uterine activity for contractions that are too frequent or too long or a uterus that does not relax for at least 30 to 60 seconds between contractions. Blood pressure and pulse identify changes from the baseline; temperature assessment identifies infection that may occur with ruptured membranes. Intake and output, assessment for headache, blurred vision, behavioral changes, increased blood pressure and respirations, decreased pulse, rales, wheezing, and coughing identify possible water intoxication. Postpartum hemorrhage may occur if an overstimulated uterus cannot contract effectively after birth.
6. In addition to identifying the true cause of the nonreassuring assessments, interventions may include stopping the oxytocin infusion, increasing the rate of the nonadditive infusion, positioning to avoid aortocaval compression, and giving oxygen by face mask. Internal monitoring may be initiated if not already in place. The physician may also order a tocolytic drug if uterine hyperactivity is the problem.
7. (a) A nonstress test evaluates placental function and apparent fetal health to avoid stressing a fetus that may already be compromised. (b) The epidural block or sedative provides pain relief for this uncomfortable procedure, although maternal discomfort would also provide a sign of problems that may indicate that the version procedure should be stopped. (c) Ultrasound guides the version and helps monitor the FHR. (d) A tocolytic drug relaxes the uterus to make the version easier to perform. (e) Administering Rh immune globulin destroys fetal Rh-positive red blood cells (RBCs) that might stimulate anti-Rh antibodies in the Rh-negative woman. These may enter the mother's bloodstream because of tiny placental disruptions during the version.

(f) FHR monitoring evaluates how the fetus is tolerating the version and when the fetal condition returns to baseline afterward. (g) Uterine activity monitoring identifies persistent contractions that may herald the onset of labor following the version.
8. (a) Add a catheter to the delivery table to empty the mother's bladder (if she is not already catheterized), making more room for the instrument-assisted birth. In the postpartum period, observe for trauma, usually lacerations (bright red bleeding with a firm fundus) or hematoma (excessive pain, edema, discoloration). Cold packs to the perineal area limit bruising and edema. (b) Observe for reddening, mild bruising, or small lacerations where forceps were applied. A chignon is typical if a vacuum extractor is used. Explain that these minor problems usually resolve quickly. Facial asymmetry, usually seen when the infant is crying, suggests nerve damage that resolves more slowly. (c) Conditions that may make a cesarean birth preferable to speed delivery or reduce trauma, such as severe fetal compromise, acute maternal conditions, high fetal station, and conflict between fetal and pelvic sizes. See also p. 371.
9. Refer to p. 373 and Chapter 17, pp. 406-407 to complete this exercise.
10. Refer to pp. 373-374 and Chapter 17, p. 404, Procedure 17-2, p. 405, to complete this exercise.
11. The infant may be born preterm if a cesarean birth is scheduled. Transient tachypnea may occur, caused by delayed absorption of lung fluid or persistent pulmonary hypertension. Injury, such as laceration or bruising, can occur.
12. (a) NPO status reduces the risk for aspiration of gastric contents if a general anesthetic becomes necessary. (b) Wedge under hip (or tilting the table) avoids aortocaval compression by the heavy uterus. (c) These tests identify reserve to tolerate blood loss, risk for poor blood clotting to control hemorrhage, and blood type for possible transfusion, and they prepare blood to be ready immediately if the need for transfusion arises. (d) Reduces risk for postpartum infection. (e) Keeps bladder out of the way of uterine incision.

Labeling

1. Refer to Figure 16-7 on p. 374 to complete this exercise.
2. Refer to Figure 16-8 on p. 378 to complete this exercise.
3. Refer to Figure 16-9 on p. 379 to complete this exercise.

Check Yourself

1, b; 2, d; 3, a; 4, c; 5, d; 6, a; 7, c; 8, b; 9, c; 10, d

Case Study

1. Postterm gestation is the probable reason for induction, although Linda is only 1 week past her estimated date of delivery. Other possible reasons might include thinning and increased dilation of the cervix that suggest that labor is near, previous large babies and the size of Linda's pelvis, characteristics of previous labors such as length. Gestational diabetes may be another factor because of Linda's large babies in the past (see Chapter 26 in text).

2. Tests for fetal lung maturity, such as the lecithin/sphingomyelin (L/S) ratio, and for presence of phosphatidylglycerol (PG) and phosphatidylinositol (PI), or other tests may be performed if there is any question about the actual gestation of the fetus. See Chapter 10 for discussion of these antepartum tests.

3. Facility guidelines should be followed. Set up as a secondary infusion, regulated by a pump; start and increase the rate slowly; and add to the primary infusion line at the lowest possible port. This technique ensures that the oxytocin can be stopped quickly if the need arises. The pump controls the infusion precisely. See also the Drug Guide: Oxytocin, p. 366. Observe the FHR and uterine activity for nonreassuring signs or uterine hyperstimulation.

4. Before the amniotomy, obtain baseline information about the FHR. Place absorbent underpads under Linda's hips. After the amniotomy, assess the FHR for at least 1 minute and report nonreassuring signs or significant changes from baseline; observe and chart the quantity, color, clarity, and odor of the amniotic fluid.

5. No change in the oxytocin is needed at this time, although amniotomy may increase contractions enough to allow a dosage reduction.

6. The oxytocin infusion should be stopped because some contractions have only a 20-second resting interval although the FHR on the monitor is within its previous range. This could exhaust the fetal oxygen reserve and lead to distress. In addition, labor is now well established and dilation is progressing, so stimulation does not appear to be warranted.

7. Actual care depends on how quickly the surgery must take place. Provide emotional support to reduce anxiety. Keep the partners together as much as possible. Provide preoperative teaching, abbreviated as necessary for the actual situation. Perform preoperative procedures such as indwelling catheter and clipping or shaving to remove abdominal hair. Explain who will be present at birth and their responsibilities. Explain recovery room care. Pad bony prominences. Secure legs with a safety strap. Tilt the table or place a wedge under one hip to avoid aortocaval compression. Apply the grounding pad and other monitors. Clean the incision line, and apply a sterile dressing.

8. Take vital signs (including pulse oximetry) every 15 minutes for 1 to 2 hours. Observe uterus for firmness and position, lochia, urine output, IV infusion, abdominal dressing, and pain-relief needs. Observe for return of motion and sensation (for regional block anesthesia) or level of consciousness (for general anesthesia or if sedative drugs were given).

Postpartum Physiologic Adaptations

Learning Activities

1. Match each term with its definition (a-h).

_____ Catabolism

_____ Dyspareunia

_____ Homan's sign

_____ Involution

_____ Kegel exercises

_____ Puerperium

_____ REEDA

_____ Stroke volume

a. Painful intercourse

b. Retrogressive changes that return the reproductive organs to their nonpregnancy states

c. Conversion of living cellular substances to simpler compounds

d. Acronym that helps assess wound healing

e. Quantity of blood ejected from the ventricle with each heartbeat

f. Calf pain that occurs when the foot is dorsiflexed

g. Period from childbirth until return of the reproductive organs to their nonpregnancy states

h. Method to increase tone of muscles around the vagina and urinary meatus

2. Describe postpartum changes in the
   a. Uterine muscle

   b. Uterine muscle cells

   c. Uterine lining

3. Describe the changes in lochia and when these occur.
   a.

   b.

   c.

4. Describe the effect of breastfeeding on
   a. Uterine involution

   b. Sexual intercourse

5. What is the significance of bradycardia during the early postpartum period?

6. What makes any pregnant or postpartum woman at risk for venous thrombosis? What factors increase this risk?

7. How does the leukocyte level change during the early postpartum period? How would a normal leukocyte level for a postpartum woman be interpreted for a nonpregnant woman?

8. Explain how a full bladder shortly after birth can lead to postpartum hemorrhage.

9. Why are postpartum women at risk for urinary tract infections?

10. When can women expect their menses to resume if they are breastfeeding? If they are not planning to breastfeed?

11. Describe the influence of the following hormones on lactation.

a. Estrogen

b. Progesterone

c. Prolactin

d. Oxytocin

12. What nursing measures help suppress lactation and manage the discomfort of breast engorgement?

13. Describe the proper technique to massage a soft fundus. How should the nurse expel clots?

14. Complete the following chart for postpartum assessments.

	Assessment	*What to Assess and Expected Findings*	*Deviations from Normal, Cause, and Nursing Actions*
Fundus			
Lochia			
Bladder			
Perineum			
Vital signs			
Breasts			
Lower extremities			

15. Write out in simple terms how you would teach a woman about each of the following postpartum comfort measures.
   a. Cold packs

   b. Perineal care

   c. Topical medications

   d. How to sit

   e. Analgesics

16. What teaching should you provide the postpartum woman to prevent constipation?

17. List signs and symptoms that the postpartum woman should report to her physician or nurse-midwife.

18. Describe additional nursing assessments and care for the woman who gave birth by cesarean.
   a. Respiratory

   b. Abdomen

   c. Intake and output

Check Yourself

1. When checking a woman's fundus 24 hours after cesarean birth of her third baby, the nurse finds her fundus at the level of her umbilicus, firm, and in the midline. The appropriate nursing action related to this assessment is to
   a. Document the normal assessment
   b. Determine when she last urinated
   c. Limit her intake of oral fluids
   d. Massage her fundus vigorously

2. A woman who is 18 hours postpartum says she is having "hot flashes" and "sweats all the time." The appropriate nursing response is to
   a. Report her signs and symptoms of hypovolemic shock
   b. Tell her that her body is getting rid of unneeded fluid
   c. Notify her nurse-midwife that she may have an infection
   d. Limit her intake of caffeine-containing fluids

3. A woman who is 3 hours postpartum has had difficulty in urinating. She finally urinates 100 mL. The initial nursing action is to
   a. Insert an indwelling catheter
   b. Have her drink additional fluids
   c. Assess the height of her fundus
   d. Chart the urination amount

4. When teaching the postpartum woman about peripads, the nurse should tell her that
   a. She can change to tampons when the initial perineal soreness goes away
   b. Pads having cold packs within them usually hold more lochia than regular pads
   c. Blood-soaked pads must be returned in a plastic bag to the hospital after discharge
   d. The pads should be applied and removed in a front-to-back direction

5. A young mother is excited about her first baby. Choose the best teaching to help her obtain adequate rest after discharge.
   a. Plan to sleep or rest any time the infant sleeps.
   b. Do all housecleaning while the infant sleeps.
   c. Cook several meals at once and freeze for later use.
   d. Tell family and friends not to visit for the first month.

6. Choose the best independent nursing action to aid episiotomy healing in the woman who is 24 hours postpartum.
   a. Antibiotic cream applications to the area three times each day
   b. Squirting warm water over the perineum after voiding or stooling
   c. Maintaining cold packs to the area at all times for the first 3 days
   d. Checking the leukocyte level daily and reporting changes

7. The nurse places one hand above the symphysis pubis during uterine massage to
   a. Make the massage more comfortable for the woman
   b. Increase the effectiveness of the procedure
   c. Help prevent the uterus from inverting
   d. Help determine the firmness of the uterus

8. A woman who is 4 hours postpartum ambulates to the bathroom and suddenly has a large gush of lochia rubra. The nurse's first action should be to
   a. Determine whether the bleeding slows to normal or remains large
   b. Observe vital signs for signs of hypovolemic shock
   c. Check to see what her previous lochia flow has been
   d. Identify the type of pain relief that was given when she was in labor

9. To help the postpartum woman avoid constipation, the nurse should teach her to
   a. Avoid intake of foods such as milk, cheese, or yogurt
   b. Take a laxative for the first 3 postpartum days
   c. Drink at least 1600 mL of non-caffeinated fluids daily
   d. Limit her walking until the episiotomy is fully healed

10. Choose the sign or symptom that the new mother should be taught to report.
    a. Occasional uterine cramping when the infant nurses
    b. Oral temperature that is 37.2° C (99° F) in the morning
    c. Descent of the fundus one fingerbreadth each day
    d. Reappearance of red lochia after it changes to serous

Developing Insight

1. You may note that some postpartum women have a urine output that is greater than their oral fluid intake. Should you be concerned? Why or why not?

2. Ask a nurse on the gynecology surgery unit what the usual time is for a woman to first urinate after surgery (if a catheter is not used). How does this time interval compare with when a postpartum woman is expected to first urinate?

3. Write a narrative nurse's note to document expected findings for a postpartum woman 12 hours after birth.

Case Study

Nita is a multipara who vaginally delivered twin boys 4 hours ago. One weighed 6 lb and the other weighed 5 lb, 6 oz. She is admitted to the mother-baby unit after an uneventful recovery. Your initial assessment reveals the following data: temperature, 37.6° C (97.9° F); pulse, 60 beats per minute (bpm); respirations 20 breaths per minute; blood pressure, 110/70 mm Hg; fundus slightly soft and located to the right of the umbilicus; lochia moderate; midline episiotomy intact with slight edema.

1. What is your interpretation of these data?

2. What is your first intervention? Why? What should you do next?

3. What should you immediately teach Nita?

Nita's vital signs 8 hours after birth are blood pressure, 112/80 mm Hg; temperature, 37.2° C (99° F); pulse, 52 bpm; and respirations, 18 breaths per minute.

4. Are any nursing interventions needed based on these vital signs? What is the rationale for your judgment?

Nita plans to breastfeed her twins. She successfully breastfed her other two children. However, she says, "I want to breast-feed, but I really have a lot of cramping when I nurse. I don't remember having that with the other two children."

5. What is the nurse's best response?

6. How should the nurse explain why Nita is having more cramping than with her other two births?

7. What intervention can help this problem?

Nita is worried about constipation because she had the problem after her previous births and has been constipated during the last months of this pregnancy.

8. What interventions and teaching can help Nita avoid constipation?

Nita will receive Rho(D) immune globulin (RhoGAM) and rubella vaccine before discharge.

9. Under what circumstances are these drugs given?

10. What precautions should the nurse teach Nita? Why?

On a clinic visit 3 days postpartum, the nurse assesses Nita's fundus as firm, midline, and 1 cm below the umbilicus.

11. Are these assessments normal? Why or why not? If they are not normal, is there an explanation?

12. What kind of lochia should the nurse expect Nita to have at this time?

Nita's episiotomy is slightly reddened along the suture line; the edges are closely approximated, and there is no edema, bruising, or drainage.

13. Do these data support the supposition that the episiotomy is healing properly? Why or why not? What nursing actions are appropriate?

ANSWERS TO SELECTED QUESTIONS

Learning Activities

1. c, a, f, b, h, g, d, e
2. (a) Stretched uterine muscle fibers contract and gradually regain their former size and contour. (b) The number of uterine muscle cells remains the same, but each cell decreases in size through catabolism. (c) The outer area of endometrium (decidua) is expelled with the placenta. Remaining decidua separates into two layers: the superficial layer is shed in lochia and the basal layer regenerates new endothelium.
3. (a) Lochia rubra contains blood, mucus, and bits of decidua; is red or red-brown; and has a duration of approximately 3 days. (b) Lochia serosa contains serous exudate, erythrocytes, leukocytes, and cervical mucus; is pinkish or brown-tinged; and its duration is from approximately the fourth to the tenth day. (c) Lochia alba contains leukocytes, decidual cells, epithelial cells, fat, cervical mucus, and bacteria; is white, yellow, or cream colored; and begins on approximately the eleventh day and may last 3 to 6 weeks.
4. (a) Breastfeeding stimulates release of oxytocin from the pituitary gland, which tends to intensify afterpains but also maintains better uterine contraction; this facilitates involution. (b) Lactation suppresses ovulation and estrogen secretion, causing more vaginal dryness than nonlactating mothers have. This may cause painful sexual intercourse unless lubrication is added.
5. Bradycardia is normal. Blood volume and cardiac output increase as blood from the uteroplacental unit returns to the central circulation and as excess extracellular fluid enters the vascular compartment for excretion. Because stroke volume increases, pulse decreases.
6. Pregnant and postpartum women have higher fibrinogen levels, which increase the ability to form clots. Factors that lyse clots are not increased, however. Women with varicose veins, a history of thrombophlebitis, or a cesarean birth have additional risks above the baseline risk.
7. Leukocytes increase up to $30,000/mm^3$, with an average of 14,000 to $16,000/mm^3$. Refer to Appendix A to answer the second question.
8. A full bladder moves the uterus out of its normal position. This interferes with the ability of the uterus to contract firmly to occlude open vessels at the placental site, allowing them to bleed freely.
9. Increased bladder capacity and decreased bladder tone along with rapid diuresis may cause urinary retention. Stasis of urine increases the risk of bacterial growth.
10. Women who are breastfeeding may not resume menses for 12 weeks to 18 months, depending on the length and frequency of breastfeeding. Lactation is not a good method of contraception, however. Women who formula feed will probably begin menses between 7 and 9 weeks postpartum.
11. (a, b) Estrogen and progesterone prepare the breasts for lactation. (c) Prolactin initiates milk production in the alveoli. (d) Oxytocin causes milk ejection from the alveoli into the lactiferous ducts.
12. Tell the mother to wear a well-fitting bra or sports bra 24 hours a day. Ice applications and analgesics reduce discomfort. She should avoid actions that stimulate milk production, such as spraying with warm water during showers and pumping or massaging the breasts.
13. Refer to Procedure 17-1 to complete this exercise.
14. Refer to text, pp. 400 and 402-406, to check your answers for this exercise.
15. The answer to this exercise should be in your own words and should fit the women you care for in your clinical setting.
16. Increase activity progressively, drink adequate fluids (at least 8 glasses of water daily), and add dietary fiber (found in fruits and vegetables, whole grain cereals, bread, and pasta) to prevent constipation. Prunes are a natural laxative.
17. Fever; localized area of redness, swelling, or pain in the breasts that is unrelieved by support or analgesics; persistent abdominal tenderness or feelings of pelvic fullness or pelvic pressure; persistent perineal pain; frequency, urgency, or burning when urinating; change in lochia character (increased amount, return to red color, passage of clots, or foul odor); localized tenderness, redness, or warmth of the legs; an abdominal incision with redness, edema, separation of edges, or foul drainage.
18. (a) If epidural narcotics were used, check the pulse oximeter or apnea monitor, or observe respiratory rate and depth every 30 minutes to 1 hour according to policy; auscultate breath sounds for retained secretions; assist the mother to turn, cough, and deep-breathe; use incentive spirometer. (b) Assess for return of peristalsis by auscultating bowel sounds; observe for abdominal distention; observe surgical dressing for intactness and drainage; observe incision line after dressing removal for signs of infection (REEDA [redness, ecchymosis, edema, drainage, approximation]); palpate fundus gently. (c) Monitor IV for rate of flow and site condition; observe urine for amount, color, and clarity.

Check Yourself

1. 1, a; 2, b; 3, c; 4, d; 5, a; 6, b; 7, c; 8, a; 9, c; 10, d

Case Study

1. Nita's fundus is not well contracted, probably because of a full bladder, because it is positioned to the right of the umbilicus. Her multifetal birth and multiparity increase the risk of postpartum hemorrhage.

2. Massage the uterus to cause it to contract firmly and control bleeding. The next intervention should be to assist Nita to empty her bladder or catheterize her (with an order) if she is unable to void. Otherwise, the uterus will relax again.

3. You should immediately teach Nita how to assess her uterus for firmness and the effect of a full bladder, her multiparity, and her multifetal birth on uterine contraction.

4. No interventions are needed. Bradycardia and a slight elevation in temperature are common at this time.

5. The nurse should reassure Nita that the afterpains are normal and are typically short-term and that analgesics can ease them. The nurse should also teach Nita that a full bladder will worsen afterpains.

6. Two factors increase afterpains in Nita's case: multiparity and uterine overdistention with two fetuses.

7. Prescribed analgesics given for postpartum discomfort will not harm the infant if taken for a short time. Lying in a prone position with a small pillow or folded blanket under the abdomen often helps.

8. Teach Nita to gradually increase her ambulation, drink additional fluids (at least 8 glasses of water daily), and increase dietary fiber. Prunes are a natural laxative, and she can consult her birth attendant for recommended laxatives if natural remedies do not work.

9. Rho(D) immune globulin is given to the Rh-negative mother if her infant is Rh-positive and if she has not previously built up anti-Rh antibodies. Rubella vaccine is given to the nonimmune postpartum woman because it is highly unlikely that she will get pregnant soon and she is then protected from the disease.

10. Nita should be cautioned to avoid another pregnancy for at least 4 weeks because a fetus may be harmed by the live virus in rubella vaccine.

11. Nita's fundus is slightly higher than usual, but this is explained by her delivery of twins.

12. Lochia flow should be rubra (possibly changing to serosa), scant, and free of foul odor or clots.

13. Slight reddening is typical of normal healing at this early stage. Close approximation of the edges and lack of drainage confirm that healing seems to be taking place normally. Proper perineal cleansing and pad application should be reinforced. The nurse should also review signs and symptoms of infection to report.

Postpartum Psychosocial Adaptations

Learning Activities

1. Match each term with its definition (a-f).

_____ Attachment

a. Position that facilitates eye-to-eye contact between parent and newborn

_____ Bonding

b. Intense fascination between father and newborn

_____ En face

c. Initial characteristic touch of mother with her newborn

_____ Engrossment

d. Development of an emotional tie to the infant

_____ Entrainment

e. Long-term development of affection between the infant and significant other

_____ Fingertipping

f. Movement of the newborn in rhythm with adult speech

2. Describe the processes of bonding and attachment. Note the similarities and differences in these processes.
   a. Bonding

   b. Attachment

3. Describe progression of maternal touch.

4. Describe progression of maternal verbal behaviors.

5. Complete the following table by describing maternal behaviors during the postpartum period. How can nurses help mothers meet their needs in each phase?

Phase	Maternal Behaviors	Nursing Considerations
Taking-in		
Taking-hold		
Letting-go		
Anticipatory stage		
Formal stage		
Informal stage		
Personal stage		
Appreciating the body		
Settling-in		
Becoming a new family		

6. Describe postpartum blues. What is the best response to the blues?

7. How can the nurse help the new father adapt to his role?

8. Describe possible responses of toddlers to a new baby. How can parents help these toddlers?

9. How should the nurse respond to the parents who are disappointed in the sex of the newborn?

10. What nursing measures can help the mother of twins attach to her babies?

11. What does "mothering the mother" entail?

12. New parents may not recognize signals from the infant that he or she has had enough stimulation and now needs to rest. What signals should the nurse teach parents to recognize?

Check Yourself

1. Twelve hours after birth, a mother lies in bed resting. Although she has only one more day in the hospital, she does not ask about her baby or provide any care. What is the probable reason for her behavior?
   a. She is still in the taking-in phase of maternal adaptation.
   b. She shows behaviors that may lead to postpartum depression.
   c. She is still affected by medications given during labor.
   d. She may be dissatisfied with some aspect of the newborn.

2. Which stage of maternal role attainment is focused on getting acquainted with the infant's individual personality?
   a. Anticipatory
   b. Formal
   c. Informal
   d. Personal

3. At her 6-week checkup, a woman expresses frustration because she is "still fat." The appropriate initial nursing response is to
   a. Explain that safe weight loss will take approximately 6 to 12 months
   b. Reassure her that she does not look fat to others
   c. Provide a low-calorie diet to help speed her weight loss
   d. Advise her to begin aerobic exercise with her diet

4. A new father is reluctant to "spoil" his newborn by picking her up when she cries. The best nursing response is to
   a. Teach him that she will eventually stop crying if he waits
   b. Take the baby to the nursery to allow the parents to rest
   c. Pick the baby up and rock her until she sleeps again
   d. Tell the father that the baby cries to communicate a need

5. A newborn is in the crib in his mother's room. The teenaged mother is watching TV. When the nurse notes that the baby is awake and quiet, the best nursing action is to
   a. Pick the baby up and point out his alert behaviors to the mother
   b. Tell the mother to pick up her baby and talk with him while he is awake
   c. Focus care on the mother, rather than the infant, so that the mother can recuperate
   d. Encourage the mother to feed the infant before he begins crying

6. The nurse can encourage the parents to care for their infant by
   a. Staying out of the room for as long as possible
   b. Having the grandmother nearby as a backup
   c. Giving positive feedback when they provide care
   d. Correcting their performance whenever they make a mistake

Developing Insight

1. If you are a parent, did you or your partner experience separation grief when it was necessary to return to work after childbirth? How did you cope with it?

2. During clinical practice, observe the reactions of siblings to a new infant. What steps do you see parents take to reassure the older child that he or she is still loved?

3. What cultural practices related to childbirth do you see in your clinical setting? Does the nursing staff support these? Discuss specific cultural practices with new parents of a different culture than your own.

4. Attend a postpartum clinic or class. Ask the parents attending what has been different (or more difficult) than they expected about the postpartum period.

5. Ask family members or friends about their experiences with postpartum blues. What was helpful and not helpful in assisting them during this time?

ANSWERS TO SELECTED QUESTIONS

Learning Activities

1. e, d, a, b, f, c
2. (a) Bonding describes the initial attraction felt by parents toward their newborn infant. It is a one-way process, from parent to infant. (b) Attachment describes a long-term, two-way process that binds parent and infant with mutual affection. Attachment is facilitated by positive feedback from the infant and by mutually satisfying experiences.
3. Maternal touch progression is from fingertipping to palm touch to enfolding the infant and bringing him or her close to the mother's body.
4. The mother progresses from calling the infant "it" to referring to the infant as "he" or "she" to using the infant's given name.
5. Refer to text, pp. 424-425, to complete this exercise.
6. Postpartum blues describes a mild, temporary depression that affects 70% to 80% of U.S. women. It begins in the first week and lasts no longer than 2 weeks. The woman has fatigue, insomnia, tearfulness, mood instability, irritability, and anxiety but is able to care for her baby. The primary nursing care is to provide empathy and support and let the woman and her family know that the condition is normal and self-limiting.
7. The nurse should involve the father in infant care teaching and decisions. Fathers may not know what to expect from newborns and benefit from information about growth and development. A review of any prenatal teaching is helpful, as well.
8. During the mother's pregnancy, toddlers may not understand that a new baby is coming. Jealousy may be shown by negative or hostile behaviors. Sleep problems and regression may also occur. Parents need to show their continued love to help the toddler understand that he or she will not be displaced by the new baby.
9. The nurse should help the parents acknowledge and talk about their feelings to help them cope with their disappointment and to facilitate their attachment with the child.
10. The nurse provides opportunities for frequent contact with each infant to help parents interact with each twin individually rather than interacting with them as a "package." It is essential to point out unique qualities and characteristics of each infant individually.
11. "Mothering the mother" involves providing physical and psychosocial care for the new mother during the early period after childbirth. The nurse should meet the physical needs, listen to the mother's concerns, and provide teaching. When the mother's needs are met, she can meet the infant's needs more easily.
12. Signs of overstimulation of the infant include looking away, splaying the fingers, arching the back, and fussiness. These are clues that the infant needs some quiet time.

Check Yourself

1, a; 2, b; 3, a; 4, d; 5, a; 6, c

Normal Newborn: Processes of Adaptation

Learning Activities

1. Match each term with its definition (a-g).

_____ Asphyxia

_____ Brown fat

_____ Jaundice

_____ Kernicterus

_____ Neutral thermal environment

_____ Nonshivering thermogenesis

_____ Surfactant

a. Slippery substance that reduces surface tension in lung alveoli

b. Permanent neurologic damage from bilirubin

c. Production of heat by use of specialized fat

d. Tissue designed for newborn heat production

e. Bilirubin staining of the skin and sclerae

f. Low blood oxygen and high blood and tissue carbon dioxide

g. Surroundings in which the infant can maintain a stable temperature with minimal oxygen consumption and a low metabolic rate

2. Explain how each factor helps the newborn initiate respirations.
   a. Chemical

   b. Mechanical

   c. Thermal

3. Why is adequate functional residual capacity in the lungs important?

4. On the drawing below, circle the fetal circulatory structures that change after birth and note how each changes. Write the factors that cause each to change.

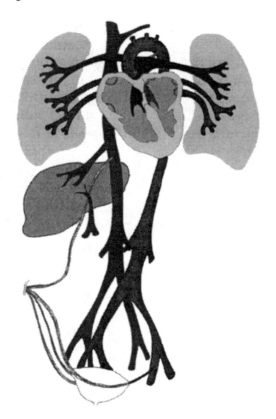

5. Number the following events in the correct order of occurrence.
_____ a. Increased blood oxygen level
_____ b. Respirations initiated
_____ c. Fibrosis of the ductus venosus
_____ d. Increased pressure in the left side of the heart
_____ e. Increased blood carbon dioxide level
_____ f. Surfactant action keeps alveoli open
_____ g. Foramen ovale closes
_____ h. Ductus arteriosus constricts

6. List characteristics that predispose newborns to heat loss.

7. Describe each method by which the newborn can lose heat. Which ones can also be methods of heat gain?

8. How does brown fat help the newborn maintain body temperature? Under what circumstances can newborns have inadequate brown fat, and why?

9. Explain the relationship between oxygenation, body temperature, glucose stores, and bilirubin levels in the newborn.

10. Compare the normal values for fetal and adult erythrocytes, hemoglobin, and hematocrit.

11. How would you explain the prophylactic neonatal vitamin K injection to new parents?

12. Describe each newborn stool as you would explain it to a new parent. When should parents expect the first meconium stool? What differences in stools should parents expect if their infant is breastfed versus formula fed?
   a. Meconium stools

   b. Transitional stools

   c. Milk stools

13. What glucose level on a screening test requires further follow-up?

14. Which infants are at risk for hypoglycemia? Why?

15. Describe how each of the following factors can contribute to high newborn bilirubin levels. Which may be correctable with nursing interventions?
   a. Red blood cell quantity and life span

   b. Liver immaturity

   c. Intestinal factors

   d. Time of first feeding, frequency of feeding

   e. Birth trauma

   f. Cold stress or asphyxia

16. When does jaundice become nonphysiologic rather than physiologic?

17. How does each of these problems result in jaundice? What is the usual treatment for each?
   a. Poor intake

   b. True breast-milk jaundice

18. Compare water distribution in the newborn and the adult.
   a. Total body water

   b. Extracellular water

19. What limitations does the newborn have in terms of
   a. Handling excess fluid

   b. Compensating for inadequate fluid

20. How much fluid does a 1-day-old newborn weighing 4082 g (9 lb) need each day?

21. What factors make the newborn vulnerable to infection that might not be a problem for an older infant or child?

22. From what pathogens does each type of antibody protect the newborn? Which ones are received from the mother?
   a. IgG

   b. IgM

   c. IgA

23. Describe the two periods of reactivity. What are the nursing implications associated with each?
   a.

   b.

24. Describe the six behavioral states seen in the newborn.
   a.

   b.

   c.

   d.

   e.

   f.

Check Yourself

1. A newborn has a hemoglobin of 24 g/dL and a hematocrit of 74%. The nurse should anticipate
   a. Temperature instability
   b. High calcium levels
   c. Delayed breastfeeding
   d. Greater than normal jaundice

2. Becoming cold can lead to respiratory distress primarily because the infant
   a. May need more oxygen than he or she can supply to generate heat
   b. Breathes more slowly and shallowly when hypothermic
   c. Reopens fetal shunts when the body temperature reaches 36.1° C (97° F)
   d. Cannot supply enough glucose to provide fuel for respirations

3. The primary purpose of surfactant is to
   a. Maintain normal blood glucose levels
   b. Keep lung alveoli partly open between breaths
   c. Inhibit excess erythrocyte production
   d. Stimulate passage of the first meconium stool

4. The foramen ovale closes because the
   a. Arterial pressures in the lungs are higher than in the body
   b. Presence of slight hypoxia and acidosis causes constriction
   c. Blood flow through it is redirected through the liver
   d. Pressure in the left atrium is higher than in the right

5. Brown fat is used to
   a. Maintain temperature
   b. Facilitate digestion
   c. Metabolize glucose
   d. Conjugate bilirubin

6. The infant of a diabetic mother is prone to hypoglycemia because
   a. Liver conversion of glycogen to glucose is sluggish
   b. Excess subcutaneous fat reduces blood flow to tissues
   c. High insulin production rapidly metabolizes glucose
   d. Vulnerability to infections increases metabolic stress

7. The primary difference between physiologic and nonphysiologic jaundice is the
   a. Number of fetal erythrocytes that are broken down
   b. Type of feeding method chosen by the mother
   c. Location of the yellow areas on the newborn's skin
   d. Time of onset and rate of rise in bilirubin levels

8. The nurse can help prevent many cases of jaundice in the breastfed infant by
   a. Giving the infant extra water between each nursing session
   b. Teaching the mother the importance of regular and adequate nursing
   c. Placing the infant under phototherapy lights prophylactically
   d. Advising the mother about suitable formulas to use if jaundice occurs

9. Signs of infection in the newborn are often subtle because
   a. Body temperature rises slowly in response to pathogens
   b. Passive antibodies from the mother fight infection early
   c. High urine output causes a lower body temperature
   d. Leukocyte response and inflammatory signs are immature

10. A hungry infant is crying vigorously. The best initial intervention is to
    a. Immediately give formula until the infant is satisfied
    b. Place the infant in a quiet, dark area, wrapped tightly
    c. Console the infant before the mother tries to feed it
    d. Instruct parents to engage the infant in eye-to-eye contact

Developing Insight

1. During clinical practice, note steps taken to conserve the newborn's body heat. Identify which method of heat loss each is designed to interrupt.

2. Use a medical dictionary or laboratory manual to distinguish between indirect and direct bilirubin tests. How would each help identify possible causes of jaundice in the newborn?

3. What is the protocol for neonatal blood glucose screening at your clinical facility?

ANSWERS TO SELECTED QUESTIONS

Learning Activities

1. f, d, e, b, g, c, a
2. (a) Decreased blood oxygen and pH and increased blood carbon dioxide stimulate the respiratory center in the medulla. Cutting the umbilical cord vessels may end the flow of a substance from the placenta that inhibits respirations. (b) Fetal chest compression during vaginal birth forces a small amount of lung fluid from the chest and draws air into the lungs when the pressure is released. (c) The sudden change in environmental temperature at birth stimulates skin sensors, which then stimulate the brain's respiratory center. Other stimuli to breathe include suctioning, drying, holding, sounds, and light.
3. Residual air in the lungs allows the alveoli to remain partly expanded after exhalation. This reduces the work necessary to expand the alveoli with each breath.
4. Refer to text, pp. 444-446, to complete this exercise.
5. a, 4; b, 2; c, 8; d, 6; e, 1; f, 3; g, 7; h, 5
6. Thin skin; blood vessels near the surface; little insulating subcutaneous white fat; heat readily transferred from internal organs to skin; greater ratio of surface area to body mass
7. *Evaporation* occurs when wet surfaces are exposed to air and the surfaces dry. *Conduction* occurs when the infant has direct contact with a cool surface or object. *Convection* refers to heat loss to air currents near the infant. *Radiation* refers to heat loss when the infant is near, but not touching, a cold surface. All methods except evaporation can also be sources of heat gain, such as contact with warm blankets or exposure to warmed air currents or heat from a radiant warmer.
8. Brown fat is metabolized to generate heat, which is transferred to the blood vessels running through it and then circulated to the rest of the body. Infants who may have inadequate brown fat include preterm infants who may not have accumulated brown fat, those with intrauterine growth restriction whose stores were depleted, and those exposed to prolonged cold stress who use up their brown fat.
9. Heat production requires oxygen for metabolism, which can exceed the infant's capacity to supply the oxygen. Cold stress decreases production of surfactant, which can cause respiratory difficulty. Glucose use is accelerated when the metabolic rate rises to produce heat, possibly depleting these stores and resulting in hypoglycemia. Metabolism of glucose and brown fat without adequate oxygen causes increased production of acids. These acids may cause jaundice because they interfere with transport of bilirubin to the liver, where it can be conjugated and excreted.
10. Values for all three are higher in the newborn than in the older infant or adult. The fetus needs these higher levels to supply adequate oxygen to the tissues because the partial pressure of oxygen in fetal blood is lower than in the adult.
11. Newborns may have a problem with bleeding because they have a temporary lack of vitamin K, which is necessary for clotting. One injection of vitamin K given shortly after birth provides the newborn with vitamin K until the intestines are able to make it.
12. Refer to p. 451 to complete this exercise.
13. Glucose lower than 40 to 45 mg/dL
14. Preterm or small-for-gestational-age infants are at risk because adequate glycogen and possibly fat may not have accumulated. Postterm infants may have used up their stores of glycogen before birth as a result of deteriorating placental function. Large-for-gestational-age infants may produce excessive insulin that quickly consumes their glucose, especially if the mother is diabetic. In addition, stress or hypothermia may consume all available glucose.
15. (a) Newborns have more erythrocytes for their size, and these break down faster than adult erythrocytes, producing a larger amount of bilirubin. (b) The liver is immature and does not immediately produce enough uridine diphosphoglucuronyl transferase to conjugate bilirubin as quickly as it is produced. (c) Lack of normal intestinal flora prevents reduction of conjugated bilirubin to urobilinogen and stercobilin for excretion. Large amounts of beta-glucuronidase in the intestines convert conjugated bilirubin back into the unconjugated form. (d) Early and frequent feedings helps establish normal intestinal flora and speeds passage of meconium. (e) Birth trauma may cause added hemolysis of erythrocytes, adding to the bilirubin load. (f) Metabolism of brown fat for heat production and asphyxia, which results in anaerobic metabolism, both produce fatty acids. The fatty acids bind more readily to albumin than bilirubin, resulting in more unconjugated and unbound bilirubin in the circulation. Cold stress can be prevented and the time of the first feeding and frequency of feedings can be altered by nursing interventions.
16. Nonphysiologic jaundice rises more rapidly and to higher levels than expected or stays elevated longer than expected. See Figure 19-7 for bilirubin levels at different times after birth.
17. (a) Inadequate intake of colostrum or formula causes retention of meconium, which is high in bilirubin. High levels of beta-glucuronidase in the intestine deconjugate bilirubin in the meconium, adding to the load on the liver. Poor intake reduces the lactating mother's milk supply, worsening the problem. Nursing measures and teaching to stimulate the infant to feed

better and, in the breastfeeding mother, increase milk production are appropriate treatment. (b) True breastmilk jaundice is characterized by rising bilirubin levels later than the first 3 to 5 days after birth that usually peak at 5 to 10 mg/dL. Jaundice can last several months. Treatment may include frequent feedings, phototherapy, formula supplementation, and possibly discontinuing breastfeeding for 12 to 48 hours.

18. (a) Water is 78% of a newborn's body but only 60% of an adult's body. (b) The proportion of extracellular water in newborns is more than double that of adults.

19. (a) A newborn's kidneys are not well equipped to handle a large load of fluid, which may cause fluid overload. (b) Newborns have half the adult's ability to concentrate urine and thus cannot conserve fluid efficiently.

20. A 1-day-old infant needs 40 to 60 mL/kg or 18 to 27 mL/lb per day. If the infant weighs 4082 g (9 lb), the infant would need 162 to 245 mL/day.

21. Leukocytes respond slowly to the site of infection and are inefficient in destroying invading organisms. The usual inflammatory response may not be present. Fever is often not present because of the immature hypothalamus.

22. (a) IgG is received from the mother to provide passive antibodies to viruses, bacteria, and bacterial toxins to which the mother has immunity. The infant increases production of his or her own IgG after 6 months of age. (b) IgM is produced by the infant to protect against gram-negative bacteria. (c) IgA is produced by the infant and is received in colostrum and breast milk. It helps protect against infections of the respiratory and gastrointestinal systems.

23. (a) Newborns during the first period of reactivity are wide awake and active. Respirations may be as high as 80 breaths per minute, and the heart rate may be as high as 180 beats per minute. Respiratory assessments show nasal flaring, crackles, retractions, and increased mucous secretions. This is an ideal time to facilitate parent-infant acquaintance, because both are highly interested in each other. (b) After the sleep period following the first period of reactivity, infants are alert, interested in feeding, and often pass meconium. The pulse and respiratory rates may increase, and some infants may have cyanosis or periods of apnea. Mucous secretions increase. The nurse must be alert for respiratory complications during this stage.

24. Refer to text, pp. 457-458, to complete this exercise.

Check Yourself

1, d; 2, a; 3, b; 4, d; 5, a; 6, c; 7, d; 8, b; 9, d; 10, c

Assessment of the Normal Newborn

Learning Activities

1. Match each term with its definition (a-h).

_____ Acrocyanosis

_____ Brick dust stain

_____ Choanal atresia

_____ Crepitus

_____ Nuchal cord

_____ Rugae

_____ Scaphoid

_____ Strabismus

a. Grating sensation during palpation

b. "Crossed" eyes

c. Bluish color of the hands and feet

d. Sunken appearance

e. Scrotal skin creases

f. Pinkish color on a wet diaper

g. Cord around the fetal neck

h. Abnormality of the nasal septum causing obstruction

2. The two immediate newborn assessments after birth are for

a.

b.

3. Complete the following table.

Head Variation	Cause(s)	Characteristic Features	Parent Teaching
Molding			
Caput succedaneum			
Cephalhematoma			

4. Explain the possible significance of each neonatal assessment.
   a. Two-vessel umbilical cord

   b. Simian crease or line

   c. Unequal gluteal creases

d. Hair tuft on lower spine

e. Ears below the level of the outer canthi of the eyes

f. Drooping of one side of the mouth

5. Complete the following table on newborn measurements.

Measurement	Average for Full-Term Infant	Possible Causes for Deviations
Weight		
Length		
Head circumference		
Chest circumference		

6. List the normal ranges for term neonatal vital signs. Describe the correct assessment technique for each.
   a. Pulse rate

   b. Respiratory rate

   c. Blood pressure

   d. Temperature
      Axillary

      Rectal

7. Why should the nurse avoid taking a rectal temperature on newborns?

8. List at least five signs that suggest neonatal respiratory distress.

9. List signs that suggest neonatal hypoglycemia.

10. Describe normal assessments of the genitalia.
   a. Female

   b. Male

11. State the possible significance of each skin variance. Note whether any special care is needed.
   a. Ruddiness

   b. Green-tinged discoloration of skin and vernix

   c. Red, blotchy areas with white or yellow papules in center

   d. Blue-black marks over the sacral area

   e. Flat, purplish area that does not blanch with pressure

   f. Red, raised, rough lesion on the head

   g. Light-brown spots

12. What facial marks may be present if the infant had a nuchal cord?

Matching

Listed are conditions that may be found when the newborn is assessed. Match the condition with the part or parts of the body where it would be observed. Note if it is found only in males or only in females. Star those that are abnormal variations.

1. _____ Candidiasis		a. Head
2. _____ Pseudomenstruation		b. Mouth
3. _____ Jaundice		c. Skin
4. _____ Engorgement		d. Genitalia
5. _____ Choanal atresia		e. Spine
6. _____ Cephalohematoma		f. Ear
7. _____ Syndactyly		g. Eye
8. _____ Preauricular sinus		h. Nose
9. _____ Hydrocele		i. Breast
10. _____ Subconjunctival hemorrhage		j. Hands and feet
11. _____ Caput succedaneum		k. Hip
12. _____ Lanugo		
13. _____ Epstein's pearls		
14. _____ Hymenal tag		
15. _____ Polydactyly		
16. _____ Developmental dysplasia		
17. _____ Spina bifida		
18. _____ Cataract		
19. _____ Hypospadias		
20. _____ Vernix caseosa		

Check Yourself

1. An infant weighing 4394 g (9 lb, 11 oz) was born vaginally. The labor nurse reports that there was shoulder dystocia at birth but that Apgar scores were 8 at 1 minute and 9 at 5 minutes. The nurse should do a focus assessment for
   a. Hip dysplasia
   b. Head molding
   c. Clavicle fracture
   d. Cephalohematoma

2. The nurse notes that the infant's feet are turned inward. The appropriate initial nursing action is to
   a. Apply a splint or harness to the feet and lower legs
   b. Notify the pediatrician or nurse-practitioner immediately
   c. Explain to the parents that this can be corrected with surgery
   d. Determine whether the feet can be moved to a normal position

3. While performing an admission assessment on a term newborn, the nurse notes poor muscle tone and slight jitteriness. There are no other findings. The appropriate nursing action is to
   a. Assess the infant's blood glucose level
   b. Wrap the infant tightly in blankets
   c. Check the chart for narcotics given in labor
   d. Give supplemental oxygen by face mask

4. When assessing a 2-day-old newborn, the nurse notes that the infant's skin color is yellowish to the level of the umbilicus. The most important action is to
   a. Teach the mother to nurse the infant at least every 2 to 3 hours
   b. Explain that jaundice is common and will resolve without treatment
   c. Ask the mother whether she has been feeding the infant supplemental formula
   d. Notify the pediatrician or nurse-practitioner of the early, intense jaundice

5. Choose the nursing observation that is most important if the nurse notes a two-vessel umbilical cord.
   a. Urine output
   b. Onset of jaundice
   c. Respiratory rate
   d. Heart rhythm

6. An infant's gestational age assessment reveals that she is SGA. This means that
   a. She was born before 37 completed weeks of gestation
   b. Her weight falls between the 10th and 90th percentile
   c. She has a low birth-weight in relation to her length
   d. Her size is smaller than expected for her gestation

7. When weighing an infant, the nurse places a covering on the scale tray to
   a. Avoid causing multiple Moro reflexes when weighing
   b. Ensure that conductive heat loss from the infant is minimal
   c. Compensate for negative weight balance to ensure correct weight
   d. Avoid contaminating the nurse's hands with body substances

8. When performing an admission assessment on a term newborn, the nurse notes that the lung sounds are slightly moist. The skin color is pink except for acrocyanosis. Pulse is 156 beats per minute and respirations are 55 breaths per minute and unlabored. The appropriate nursing action is to
   a. Notify the pediatrician of the abnormal lung sounds
   b. Continue to observe the infant's respiratory status
   c. Recheck the high respiratory and pulse rates in 30 minutes
   d. Keep the infant in the newborn nursery until stable

9. To elicit the Babinski reflex the nurse should
   a. Place a finger at the base of the infant's toes and press gently
   b. Begin at the middle toe and stroke down the center of the foot
   c. Stroke the lateral sole from the heel up and across the ball of the foot
   d. Stroke across the dorsal aspect of the toes to the center of the foot

10. The best location for an infant's glucose determination is the
    a. Great toe of either foot
    b. Nondominant heel
    c. Midline of the heel
    d. Lateral surface of the heel

Developing Insight

1. Find infants whose gestational age assessments were large for gestational age (LGA) or small for gestational age (SGA). Look at the mothers' charts to determine possible causes. Check the infants' charts to identify nursing assessments and care that were different (or more in-depth) for these infants during the early hours after birth. Did any problems develop related to their being LGA or SGA?

2. Perform a gestational age assessment on an infant. Ask a classmate to assess the infant separately. Compare your scores and discuss reasons for any differences. Do the same with a staff nurse. Be careful not to stress the infant.

3. Identify different periods of reactivity in infants. Note the response of mothers to the different periods. Determine the mothers' understanding of each period of reactivity and teach them as needed.

4. Identify habituation and self-consoling activities in infants. Determine what stimuli caused the habituation.

Case Study

You are admitting a newborn and performing a gestational age assessment. The infant weighs 3 kg (6 lb, 10 oz); her length is 48.25 cm (19 in); her head circumference is 33 cm (13 in). You obtain this information on the assessment: fully flexed position; 0-degree wrist angle; 90- to 100-degree angle on arm recoil; 90-degree popliteal angle; elbow reaches sternum when extending arm across the chest; lower leg at 90-degree angle when flexing thigh onto abdomen. Skin is dry and cracking and no blood vessels are visible through the skin. Little lanugo is present. Sole creases cover the entire foot. Areola is 4 mm and ear cartilage is stiff. Clitoris and labia minora are completely covered by the labia majora.

1. Using Figure 20-19, circle the previous information on the neuromuscular and physical maturity scale. What is your total score for both?

2. Determine the approximate weeks of gestation.

3. Using Figure 20-31, plot the infant's weight, length, and head circumference. Determine whether she is SGA, appropriate for gestational age (AGA), or LGA.

4. Based on your assessments, does the nurse need additional care for this infant? Why or why not?

ANSWERS TO SELECTED QUESTIONS

Learning Activities

1. c, f, h, a, g, e, d, b
2. (a) Respiratory problems; (b) obvious anomalies
3. Refer to text, pp. 469-470, to complete this exercise.
4. (a) Associated with other anomalies; assess infant carefully. (b) Single palmar crease that often occurs in infants who have chromosomal abnormalities such as Down syndrome. (c) Suggests one leg is shorter than the other; often associated with developmental hip dysplasia. (d) May indicate spina bifida occulta, or failure of one or more vertebrae to close fully. (e) Associated with chromosomal disorders. (f) Indicates facial nerve injury during birth resulting in paralysis.
5. Refer to Table 20-1 to complete this exercise.
6. Refer to text, pp. 467-468, and Procedure 20-1 to complete this exercise.
7. Taking a rectal temperature on newborns may irritate the mucosa or perforate the rectum, which turns at a right angle 3 cm (1.2 inches) from the anal sphincter.
8. (In any order) (a) tachypnea (sustained); (b) retractions that continue after the first hour; (c) nasal flaring after the first hour; (d) cyanosis involving the lips, tongue, and trunk (central cyanosis); (e) grunting; (f) seesaw respirations; (g) asymmetry of chest expansion
9. Jitteriness, poor muscle tone, sweating, respiratory signs (dyspnea, apnea, cyanosis, tachypnea, grunting), low temperature, poor suck, high-pitched cry, lethargy, seizures, eventually coma; some show no signs of hypoglycemia
10. (a) Labia majora darker than surrounding skin and completely covering the clitoris and labia minora; white mucous discharge or pseudomenstruation; hymenal or vaginal tags; patent urinary meatus and vagina. (b) Pendulous scrotum that is darker than surrounding skin and covered with rugae; testes palpable in the scrotal sac; meatus centered at the tip of the glans penis; prepuce covering the glans and adherent to it.
11. (a) Suggests polycythemia; may cause higher bilirubin levels as the excessive erythrocytes break down, so observe for more severe jaundice and emphasize to parents. (b) Indicates meconium passage in utero; observe infant for associated respiratory difficulties resulting from aspirated meconium. (c) Erythema toxicum; differentiate from infection; teach parents that rash is self-limiting. (d) Mongolian spots; more common in dark-skinned infants; most disappear during early years; teach parents who are unfamiliar with these. (e) Nevus flammeus (port-wine stain); permanent; large or obvious ones can later be removed by laser surgery. (f) Nevus vasculosus (strawberry hemangioma); grows larger for 5 to 6 months, then gradually disappears. (g) Café-au-lait spots; 6 or more spots or spots larger than 0.5 cm are associated with neurofibromatosis and should be reported to the physician.
12. Petechiae on the face or upper body are often present when the infant had a nuchal cord at birth.

Matching

1, *b; 2, d (females); 3, c, g (sclera), *abnormal if present before 24 hours; 4, i; 5, *h; 6, a; 7, *j; 8, *f; 9, *d (males); 10, g; 11, a; 12, c (*suggests infant is preterm if excessive); 13, b; 14, d (females); 15, *j; 16, *k; 17, *e; 18, *g; 19, *d (males); 20, c (*suggests infant is preterm if excessive)

Check Yourself

1, c; 2, d; 3, a; 4, d; 5, a; 6, d; 7, b; 8, b; 9, c; 10, d

Case Study

1. Total maturity score is 43.
2. The infant's maturity rating is between 40 and 42 weeks (approximately 41 weeks).
3. Weight is 3000 g; length is 48.25 cm; head circumference is 33 cm. The infant is appropriate for gestational age (AGA) in all measurements.
4. All measurements fall near the 25th percentile, which means that 74% of infants of this gestational age are larger and 24% are smaller. The infant is AGA. The nurse would not anticipate the need for expanded assessments or care based on the gestational age assessment alone.

Care of the Normal Newborn

Common Concerns of Students Teaching Parents

Students without newborn experience often worry about their ability to teach new parents. Concerns include lack of experience, fear of giving inaccurate information, and dealing with experienced mothers. However, there are many methods for increasing knowledge and confidence to make parent teaching one of the most enjoyable aspects of nursing.

Resources

Take advantage of available resources for increasing your knowledge of infant care. In addition to reading nursing textbooks, visit college and hospital libraries for journal articles about newborn nursing care. Parent education materials available on the maternity unit or on the Internet provide easy-to-read, quick information.

Seek out resource people who can help. Most nurses enjoy sharing their knowledge. To learn teaching approaches and answers to common parent questions, listen as they work with parents. Talk to the lactation consultant to learn more about breastfeeding. Attend parent classes on infant care and feeding.

Make use of audiovisual materials for parent education. Watching a DVD with parents helps the student and parents learn and provides a starting place for clarifying parent questions.

Repetitive Teaching

Students have the opportunity to repeat teaching because all parents need the same basic information. Material that is at first new quickly becomes familiar with repeat practice. Students soon become polished and develop creative new ways to present information.

Experienced Mothers

What does one teach the mother having her second (or eighth) baby? Begin by assessing the mother's knowledge. If her youngest child is older than a year or two, she has probably forgotten some of the details of infant care. Briefly review the material that is routinely given to first-time mothers to discover any gaps in the experienced mother's knowledge. For example, the mother of girls may need information about care of the penis if she has a boy. Some mothers may not know that the recommended position for sleeping infants is supine and that this helps prevent sudden infant death syndrome (SIDS).

As you teach, acknowledge the mother's past experience. For example, you may say, "I'm sure you know much of this information, but let's check this list to see whether anything has changed or you think of any questions." Insert phrases such as, "As you remember…" or "And you probably know about…" This recognizes the mother's knowledge, but allows her to refresh her memory.

Some mothers hesitate to ask about topics they think the nurse might expect them to know. Reviewing all material allows the mother to ask questions without feeling foolish. Providing an environment that is warm and accepting helps her feel it is "safe" to ask questions.

Ask the mother about her opinions and the problems she had in the past. For example, "What is the hardest part about taking care of a new baby, in your experience?" Not only does this provide an opportunity for discussion, but you may also learn from the mother's experience!

Sometimes the mother is more concerned about her other children than about the new baby. She may wonder how they will feel about the newborn and how she can meet the needs of each child when she is so tired. Use therapeutic communication techniques to act as a "sounding board" as she sorts out priorities and makes plans.

Experienced Nurse-Parents

Nursing students who are parents may rely on personal experience in parent teaching. However, personal experiences should seldom be shared with clients. Clients want to talk about their own situation and may not believe that the nurse's experiences apply. In addition, information about infant care changes. Nurses who rely on their own parenting experiences can pass along incorrect information or information that conflicts with that taught by the birth center.

Learning Activities

1. The correct order for suctioning an infant's airway with the bulb syringe is to suction the
_____ first and the _____ second. Why?

2. Why is it particularly important that the infant's head be dried promptly?

3. What added assessments and interventions should the nurse perform if an infant has a subnormal temperature?

4. What type of heat loss can occur in each situation?
   a. Placing the newborn on a cold, unpadded surface

   b. Using a cold stethoscope to listen to breath sounds

   c. Placing the infant's crib by a window on a snowy day

   d. Partially drying the infant's hair after the bath

e. Placing the infant's crib near an air conditioner vent

f. Forgetting to turn the radiant warmer on before placing the infant under it

5. A newborn who is large for gestational age (LGA) has a low blood glucose on the first screening and will need more glucose screenings until the level is stable. Explain in simple terms, as you would explain to parents, the reason for feeding the newborn promptly and for repeat screenings.

6. Explain to parents why it is important for their infant who is jaundiced to eat frequently and adequately.

7. What should the nurse teach new parents about infant
   a. Burping

   b. Urination

   c. Stools

8. What are the three primary nursing observations after circumcision?

9. What circumcision problems should parents be taught to report?

10. List signs that suggest infection at the umbilical cord. What measures can prevent cord infection?

11. What is the primary method of identifying the newborn and mother (or other support person)?

12. What are some examples of suspicious behavior in a visitor that should cause the nurse to think about the possibility of abduction?

13. List five general signs of newborn infection.
   a.

   b.

   c.

   d.

   e.

14. Explain why these medications are typically given to newborns. Which is required by state law?
   a. Vitamin K

   b. Erythromycin eye ointment

   c. Hepatitis B immunization

15. Do infants of mothers with hepatitis B need any additional medication? Why?

Check Yourself

1. An infant's axillary temperature is 35.9° C (96.6° F). The priority nursing action is to
    a. Recheck the infant's temperature rectally
    b. Have the mother breastfeed the infant
    c. Place the infant in a radiant warmer
    d. Chart the normal axillary temperature

2. To care for the uncircumcised penis, parents should be taught to
    a. Retract the foreskin with each diaper change
    b. Wash under the foreskin as far as it will retract when the child is older
    c. Use an emollient cream to hasten foreskin separation
    d. Avoid putting soap on the foreskin before separation

3. A nursing student has been caring for a woman and her newborn all morning. The student takes the infant to the nursery for screening tests before discharge. When the infant is returned to the mother, the correct procedure is to
    a. Have the mother read her printed band number and verify that it matches the infant's
    b. Ask the mother to state her name and the name of her infant
    c. Call out the mother's full name before leaving the infant with her
    d. Explain the screening tests and give the infant to the mother

4. The correct site for injection of hepatitis B immunization for a newborn is the
    a. Subcutaneous tissue of the thigh
    b. Dorsogluteal muscle
    c. Deltoid muscle
    d. Vastus lateralis muscle

5. A new mother should be taught to support her baby's head when holding the infant because
    a. Doing so will promote better eye contact and bonding
    b. The baby's muscles are too weak to support the heavy head
    c. It allows better guidance of the head toward the breast
    d. Less regurgitation of gastric contents will occur

6. A new mother anxiously summons the nurse to her room because the baby sneezed twice. A brief assessment shows nothing unusual. The appropriate teaching is that
    a. This may indicate overstimulation and the infant may need a quiet time
    b. Multiple sneezes are characteristic of the second period of reactivity
    c. The baby may be developing a cold, so the pediatrician will be notified
    d. Sneezing may indicate sensitivity to the drugs given to the mother during labor

7. Choose the normal circumcision assessment.
    a. Plastibell positioned well down the shaft of the penis
    b. Oozing of blood from the site after a Gomco circumcision
    c. Delay in urination for 12 to 16 hours after the procedure
    d. Development of a dry yellow crust on the circumcision site

8. Choose the correct parent teaching about cord care.
    a. Fold the diaper below the cord to speed drying.
    b. Expect the cord to detach in no more than 7 days.
    c. Scrub the area with soap each day.
    d. Skin near the cord site may be red until it detaches.

9. The nurse should teach the parents to position the infant's hospital crib
   a. Next to the windows to be exposed to the sun
   b. Near the mother's bed on the side opposite the door
   c. At the foot of the bed so the mother can get out of bed easily
   d. Near the door of the bathroom next to the sink

10. The nurse notes an infant sleeping on the back in the crib in the mother's room. The nurse should
    a. Turn the infant to the side to avoid aspiration from regurgitation
    b. Suggest the mother hold the infant to enhance bonding
    c. Commend the mother for positioning the infant correctly
    d. Explain the importance of the prone position for sleep

Developing Insight

1. Newborn circumcision is a controversial topic. Consider common reasons for having the procedure performed on a newborn and refute each. Do the same for reasons against having circumcision performed.

2. What screening tests are routinely performed at your clinical facility? What information is given to parents about testing?

3. What is the policy in your facility for infants with risk factors for or signs of hypoglycemia?

4. What security measures are used at your clinical facility to prevent infant abduction? Ask several parents who have previously been taught security measures to restate these measures. How well do they recall them?

5. Does your clinical facility offer follow-up care, such as warm lines, postpartum clinics, or home visits for new parents? Ask staff members about the effectiveness of such measures.

ANSWERS TO SELECTED QUESTIONS

Learning Activities

1. Mouth; nose (only if needed). The infant might gasp when the nose is suctioned, drawing any secretions that are in the mouth into the airway.
2. The head makes up a large part of the newborn's body and thus is a large surface for heat loss. Damp hair presents a continuing source for evaporative heat loss.
3. Assess for and correct sources of heat loss, such as wet clothing, drafts, or exposed skin. Place the infant skin-to-skin with the mother or wrap the flexed infant snugly in warm blankets. Apply a hat and a shirt, and use another shirt with the sleeves over the legs. A radiant warmer, regulated by a skin probe, may be needed for very low temperatures. Have the mother breastfeed or feed the infant formula if it is near feeding time. Teach parents about maintaining the infant's temperature, particularly if their actions have contributed to the low temperature.
4. (a) Conduction; (b) conduction; (c) radiation; (d) evaporation; (e) convection; (f) conduction
5. Refer to text discussion of glucose, pp. 506–507, to formulate your parent teaching.
6. Infants who do not eat well will be slower in passing stools in which bilirubin is eliminated. When feces remain in the intestines, an enzyme (beta-glucuronidase) that was important during fetal life may change the bilirubin back to a form (unconjugated) that cannot be eliminated in the stools. The bilirubin may be absorbed back into the bloodstream and the liver will have added work in changing it back to a form in which it can be excreted.
7. (a) Burp about midway through each feeding by holding the baby upright against your shoulder or in a sitting position on your lap with the head and chest supported while you pat the back. (b) The baby will have at least 1 to 2 wet diapers per day on the first day or two, increasing to at least 6 wet diapers by the fourth day. Notify the physician if there are no wet diapers in 12 hours. (c) The first stools are called meconium (tarry, greenish-black, and sticky), followed by transitional stools, followed by milk stools. The stools of breastfed babies are mustard-yellow, soft, and seedy and have a sweet-sour smell. Stools of formula-fed babies are pale yellow to light brown and formed. The baby is not constipated unless the stools are hard and dry like marbles. A water ring around the stool in the diaper indicates diarrhea and should be reported to the physician.
8. Bleeding, urination, and infection

9. Notify physician if there is no urinary output within 6 to 8 hours, bleeding more than a few drops with first diaper changes, or displacement of the Plastibell. Apply pressure if any bleeding occurs. Report signs of infection, such as redness, edema, tenderness, and discharge (a yellow exudate that dries is normal).
10. Signs of infection include redness or edema at the cord base and purulent drainage. Keep the cord area dry by folding the diaper below the area. Check with the health care provider regarding tub bathing before the cord has detached and the area is fully healed. Care generally includes cleaning the cord with water if necessary and allowing it to dry naturally.
11. Identification is accomplished by matching the imprinted numbers on the adult's wristband with those on the infant's identification bands. The numbers should be matched *every* time the infant is reunited with the parent. The nurse should visually match the numbers or have the parent or support person read the imprinted numbers from his or her band.
12. Visitors who go from one room to another, visitors who ask many questions regarding hospital routines and floor plan (exits, etc.), anyone carrying an infant in the hallway or taking a crib to areas where it should not be taken, anyone carrying a bag or package large enough to hide an infant
13. (a) Low temperature; (b) lethargy; (c) poor feeding; (d) periods of apnea without obvious cause; (e) any unexplained change in behavior; (f) drainage from the eyes, cord, or circumcision
14. (a) Vitamin K, which is necessary for normal blood coagulation, is given because the infant's gastrointestinal tract is sterile at birth and temporarily lacks the microorganisms that will make this vitamin. (b) Erythromycin ointment is required by state law to prevent eye infections acquired in the mother's birth canal, such as gonorrhea and *Chlamydia*. (c) Hepatitis B immunization is given to promote the infant's manufacture of antibodies against this viral infection of the liver.
15. Mothers who are positive for hepatitis B (carriers) may transmit the organism to their infant at birth. The first dose of a series of three doses of vaccine is given within 12 hours of birth to infants of mothers who are hepatitis carriers. These infants also receive hepatitis B immune globulin to provide passive antibody protection until the infant manufactures his or her own active antibodies to the virus.

Check Yourself

1, c; 2, b; 3, a; 4, d; 5, b; 6, a; 7, d; 8, a; 9, b; 10, c

Infant Feeding

Learning Activities

1. Match each term with its definition (a-e).

_____ Colostrum   a. Higher-fat milk

_____ Foremilk   b. Precedes true milk

_____ Hindmilk   c. Breast inflammation

_____ Mastitis   d. Allows milk to "let down"

_____ Milk-ejection reflex   e. Thirst-quenching milk

2. a. Determine the number of calories per day needed by a 3-day-old infant weighing 3.6 kg (8 lb).

b. Calculate the number of ounces of breast milk or formula (each having 20 calories per ounce) the infant needs daily.

c. What are the infant's daily fluid needs?

3. Describe changes in composition and appearance of colostrum, transitional milk, and mature milk.
   a. Colostrum

   b. Transitional milk

   c. Mature milk

4. Determine what advantages the breastfed infant receives that the formula-fed infant does not receive regarding the following components.

Component	Quantity and Advantages
Proteins	
Carbohydrates	
Fats	
Vitamins	
Minerals	
Enzymes	

5. List factors and describe the purpose of factors in breast milk that help prevent infant infections.

6. Describe the purposes of prolactin and oxytocin in breastfeeding. What can enhance or interfere with their secretion?
   a. Prolactin

   b. Oxytocin

7. What care can help the mother who has flat or inverted nipples? Are any precautions needed?

8. Describe differences in breast fullness.
   a. Soft

   b. Filling

   c. Engorged

9. Describe each of these hand positions for breastfeeding.
   a. Palmar or U position

   b. Scissors or V position

10. Describe useful techniques to teach the mother if the infant seems to have trouble breathing while nursing.

11. Describe differences between nutritive and nonnutritive suckling. How does infant swallowing sound?
   a. Nutritive

   b. Nonnutritive

   c. Swallowing

12. What should the mother be taught about burping the infant?
   a. When to burp

   b. Removing the infant from breast

13. How can you tell whether the infant needs more of the areola in the mouth? How much areola should be inside?

14. How does frequent breastfeeding help resolve jaundice?

15. List methods to prevent and treat engorgement.
   a. Prevention

   b. Treatment

16. In what maternal conditions is breastfeeding not advised?

17. What should the mother be taught about storage of breast milk?
   a. Containers

   b. Temperature

   c. Thawing frozen milk

18. How long should a mother breastfeed?

19. Describe use and precautions associated with each type of formula.
   a. Ready-to-use

   b. Concentrated liquid

   c. Powdered

20. Explain what a new mother should be taught about each of these aspects of formula feeding.
   a. Frequency

   b. Propping the bottle

   c. Microwaving formula

   d. Feeding leftover formula

Check Yourself

1. A breastfeeding mother is encouraged to nurse her infant 30 minutes after birth. The infant is awake, licks her nipple, and makes occasional suckling efforts, but does not latch on. The mother says, "Maybe I should just bottle-feed him, since he doesn't want to nurse." The best reply should emphasize that
   a. Formula feeding is usually much easier than breastfeeding
   b. The infant's actions suggest that her nipples may be too firm
   c. Breast milk production is stimulated by these early actions
   d. She will be unable to establish lactation unless the baby nurses early

2. A new mother wants to nurse her infant only 5 minutes at each breast to avoid sore nipples. Choose the appropriate teaching.
   a. Keeping early feedings short lessens nipple trauma and helps toughen nipples.
   b. Very short feedings reduce hindmilk and may interfere with the infant's weight gain.
   c. Limiting time at the breast does not reduce sore nipples but does reduce engorgement.
   d. Delay in the transition from colostrum to true milk will result from this practice.

3. A new mother wants to breastfeed, but plans occasional formula feedings. The nurse should teach her to
   a. Avoid using bottles for 3 to 4 weeks to establish her milk supply if possible
   b. Make a clear choice to feed by one method to avoid nipple confusion
   c. Limit formula feeding to once each day until her milk supply is well established
   d. Alternate formula and nursing to allow the infant to become accustomed to both

4. A woman has had a baby at 29 weeks of gestation. She tells the nurse that she cannot breastfeed because the baby is so small. The nurse should tell her that
   a. She will be able to establish lactation when the baby is strong enough to nurse
   b. Special formulas are actually better than breast milk for preterm infants
   c. Infections are more likely to occur if the infant takes stored breast milk
   d. She can use a breast pump to maintain lactation until nursing is possible

5. A breastfeeding mother is reluctant to take a prescribed analgesic because she does not want to pass it to the baby. The nurse should teach her that
   a. Medications prescribed for postpartum discomfort are safe for use in lactation
   b. She should feed less often so she can limit transfer of medication to the baby
   c. It is essential to avoid all nonessential medications during nursing, including analgesics
   d. Formula feeding as long as she needs analgesics may be best for the baby

6. The maximum length of time formula should be kept in a refrigerator after preparation is
   a. 12 hours
   b. 24 hours
   c. 36 hours
   d. 48 hours

7. A new mother is worried because her 1-day-old baby is taking only ¾ to 1 oz of formula at most feedings. The nurse should teach her that
   a. Her baby should be taking 3 to 4 oz at each feeding by the next day
   b. The amount the baby is taking at each feeding is normal at this time
   c. The baby might take more if she tries using a different formula
   d. The nipple may be too firm for the baby to suck easily and should be changed

8. A woman with active herpes asks whether she can breastfeed her infant. The nurse should tell her that
   a. She can breastfeed the infant if she does not have any lesions on her breasts
   b. She should not breastfeed the infant because the virus can infect the infant
   c. She can breastfeed after the infant has received vaccination against herpes
   d. The infant has antibodies against herpes and is unlikely to become infected

9. Which is true about breastfeeding?
   a. Immigrant women are more likely than women born in this country to breastfeed.
   b. African-American women have the highest rates of breastfeeding.
   c. Some women do not feed their infants colostrum because they think it is "spoiled."
   d. American-born women are the most likely to combine breastfeeding and formula feeding.

10. For the cross-cradle hold, the mother holds the infant's head
    a. At the antecubital space with the body along the arm and holds the breast with the other hand on the other side.
    b. In the hand on the side of the breast being used with the infant's body along her side and holds the breast with the other hand.
    c. And body close to her and facing the breast as the mother lies on her side. Pillows help position the mother and infant.
    d. In the hand opposite from the breast being used with the body across her lap and holds the breast with the other hand.

Developing Insight

1. Ask women you care for during clinical experience what their reasons were for choosing their method of feeding. Were any of their reasons based on cultural influences?

2. Use the LATCH scoring tool to assess breastfeeding mothers and infants you care for during clinical.

3. Make a teaching plan to help mothers with the following breastfeeding problems
   a. Engorgement
   b. Sore nipples
   c. Flat or inverted nipples
   d. Sleepy baby or one who falls asleep soon after nursing begins

4. A mother tells you that she does not think she has enough milk for her baby. How can you guide her?

5. If your clinical experience includes postpartum clinic or home visits, ask breastfeeding mothers whether they have encountered problems since they were discharged. If they have stopped breastfeeding, why? Have any of the women forgotten information that was taught when they were in the birth center?

6. Attend a breastfeeding class or a breastfeeding support group to learn what help is available for mothers and what they learn there.

Case Study

Margaret is breastfeeding for the first time. She seems awkward in handling her baby and says that the baby is not feeding well. The baby cries frequently while Margaret tries to feed her.

1. What is the first nursing action to take in this situation?

2. What additional nursing actions can help Margaret?

After your nursing actions, the infant latches onto the breast and begins suckling vigorously. Margaret begins to relax. She says, "I thought this would be easy, but it isn't." After about 3 minutes, Margaret asks, "Shouldn't I change breasts now? I don't want to have sore nipples."

3. Discuss the following topics with Margaret.
   a. Duration of feeding
   b. Removing the infant from the breast
   c. Frequency of feedings

4. What should you tell her about caring for her breasts?

Margaret successfully completes her first breastfeeding. She asks, "The baby seemed to suck a lot, but how do I know she is getting enough to eat?"

5. What infant signs or behaviors can you teach Margaret to look for that indicate adequate milk intake?

ANSWERS TO SELECTED QUESTIONS

Learning Activities

1. b, e, a, c, d

2. (a) If calculated using kilograms: 360 to 396 calories/day (3.6 kg × 100 calories/kg = 360; or 3.6 kg × 110 calories/kg = 396). If calculated using pounds: 360 to 400 calories/day (8 lb × 45 calories/lb = 360; or 8 lb × 50 calories/lb = 400). (b) The infant needs 18 to 20 oz of breast milk or formula daily (360, 396, or 400 divided by 20 calories/oz = 18, 19.8, or 20 oz). (c) If calculated using kilograms: 360 to 540 ml/day (3.6 kg × 100 ml/kg = 360; 3.6 kg × 150 ml/kg = 540). If calculated using pounds: 360 to 544 ml/day (8 lb × 45 ml/lb = 360 ml/day; 8 lb × 68 ml/lb = 544 ml/day).

3. (a) Colostrum is produced during the first 7 to 10 days; it is a thick, yellow substance that is rich in immunoglobulins, especially IgA. It has laxative effects and is high in protein, fat-soluble vitamins, and minerals. It is lower in carbohydrates, fat, lactose, and some vitamins than mature milk. (b) Transitional milk is lower in immunoglobulins and proteins but higher in lactose, fat, and calories than colostrum. (c) Mature milk begins after 2 weeks of lactation; it is bluish and provides 20 calories/oz. Immunoglobulins are provided in mature milk throughout lactation.

4. Refer to text, pp. 527-528, to complete this exercise.

5. Bifidus factor promotes growth of *Lactobacillus bifidus,* which increases acidity in the gastrointestinal tract. Leukocytes (macrophages) secrete lysozyme, which acts against gram-positive and enteric bacteria. Lactoferrin inhibits growth of iron-dependent bacteria. Immunoglobulins, particularly IgA, help protect against gastrointestinal and ear infections.

6. (a) Prolactin stimulates the breasts to produce milk. It is enhanced by suckling and removal of milk from the breasts. It is inhibited by estrogen, progesterone, and placental lactogen during pregnancy and by inadequate removal of milk after nursing begins. (b) Oxytocin stimulates the milk-ejection reflex. It is enhanced by comfort, thinking about the infant, and the stimulation of suckling. It is inhibited by discomfort or inadequate suckling.

7. Rolling flat nipples stimulates them to become more erect. Pumping breasts for a few minutes before nursing or using a breast shield draws inverted nipples out so that the infant can grasp them. Breast shells used in late pregnancy or between feedings to help draw nipples out are controversial. Stretching or other manipulation of the nipples is unnecessary and should be avoided during pregnancy because it may cause uterine contraction.

8. (a) Feel like a cheek; (b) slightly firmer than a cheek; (c) hard, shiny, taut tissue

9. (a) The mother cups the breast in her palm with her thumb on top and the fingers underneath and behind the areola. (b) In the scissors or V position, the mother places her index and middle finger above and beneath the areola to guide her nipple to the infant.

10. The mother can bring the infant into a more horizontal position and nearer her body. She should not indent the breast tissue, because this may interfere with milk flow or change the position of the nipple in the infant's mouth and may lead to sore nipples.

11. (a) Nutritive suckling is evidenced by smooth, continuous movements with occasional pauses to rest. Swallowing may follow each suck or after 2 or 3 sucks. (b) Nonnutritive suckling produces fluttery or choppy motions without the sound of swallowing. (c) Infant swallowing has a soft "ka" or "ah" sound.

12. (a) For breastfeeding, burp when nonnutritive suckling begins and change to the other breast. For formula feeding, burp after approximately one-half ounce of formula in the early days, and then to midway in the feeding when the infant's intake increases. (b) Break suction before removing the infant from the breast by inserting a finger between the infant's gums or indenting the breast tissue near the infant's mouth.

13. The infant's cheeks will show dimpling, and he or she will make smacking or clicking sounds. The infant's lips should be 1 to 1½ inches from the base of the nipple if there is enough of the areola in the mouth.

14. Frequent breastfeeding enhances milk production and stimulates peristalsis, which increases the number of stools and thus helps the body excrete bilirubin.

15. (a) Early and frequent nursing for adequate lengths of time day and night helps prevent engorgement. Avoiding formula or water supplements causes the infant to eat more often than if formula is used. (b) Treatment includes feeding every 1½ to 2 hours; cold applications between feedings; heat application shortly before feeding; massage to speed milk release; softening the areola by using a pump or expressing milk to begin flow. Give medication for discomfort; advise mother to wear a well-fitting (but not tight) bra 24 hours a day.

16. Serious infections such as untreated tuberculosis, HIV infection, galactosemia, and maternal chemotherapy. Maternal substance abuse is usually also a contraindication to breastfeeding.

17. (a) Glass, polyethylene, or polypropylene plastic containers. (b) Milk can be stored in the refrigerator for 72 hours or in the freezer of a refrigerator for 1 month; it can be kept in a deep freeze at −20° C (−4° F) for 3 to 4 months. (c) Do not microwave. Thaw in the refrigerator or by holding under running water.

18. The American Academy of Pediatrics and American Dietetics Association recommend breast milk only for infants during the first 6 months. Although solid foods are added at approximately 6 months, the suggestion is for breastfeeding to continue for at least 1 year. However, the decision of how long to breastfeed is up to the mother.

19. (a) Open the bottle and add a cap for single-serving containers. For multi-serving cans, wash the top of the can and the can opener just before opening and shake the can. Pour into washed bottles and cap. Do not dilute. Refrigerate an open can and discard any remaining milk after 48 hours. (b) Dilute the concentrated liquid with an equal part of water. Do not over- or under-dilute. Fill clean bottles with diluted formula as in ready-to-feed. (c) Dilute formula in a clean bottle exactly as directed, usually one scoop for each 2 oz of water. As in concentrated liquid formula, do not over- or under-dilute.

20. (a) Feed the infant every 3 to 4 hours, following the infant's hunger cues instead of a rigid schedule. (b) Do not prop the bottle. Propping can cause aspiration of formula and increases the incidence of ear infections and dental caries (when the primary teeth erupt). (c) Do not microwave formula, because it may have "hot spots" that would burn the infant. (d) Discard all remaining formula after 1 hour of use.

Check Yourself

1, c; 2, b; 3, a; 4, d; 5, a; 6, d; 7, b; 8, a; 9, c; 10, d

Case Study

1. A good initial action would be to help Margaret calm her fussy baby so that the infant will be more likely to nurse. This action accomplishes two goals: (1) it helps Margaret learn the skill of comforting her infant, and (2) it increases the likelihood that the infant will nurse well when positioned properly at the breast.

2. After the infant is calmer, suggest positions that Margaret might use to begin nursing. Support her arm in the chosen position with pillows or blankets. Explain the basics of helping her infant latch on to the breast: stimulating the infant's mouth until it opens wide, then drawing the infant close; inserting the nipple and areola well back into the mouth; checking to see that the lips are flared on the breast tissue. Describe and have Margaret observe for typical patterns that indicate nutritive suckling: smooth rhythmic suckling, interrupted by swallowing with a soft "ka" or "ah" sound.

3. a. Teach Margaret that the milk-ejection reflex can take as long as 5 minutes to occur and nursing periods that are too short will provide only the foremilk, which has a lower fat content, is less satisfying, and does not promote the infant's growth. If the infant receives only the foremilk regularly, she will want to nurse often and will be less satisfied. Engorgement is also more likely. Duration is generally at least 10 to 15 minutes on each breast.

   b. Teach her to break the suction by inserting a finger between the infant's gums before removing the infant from the breast.

   c. Infants usually feed every 2 to 3 hours, and the mother should plan on nursing 8 to 12 times in each 24-hour period.

4. Wear a well-fitting bra day and night. Avoid creams, ointments, or soaps on the breasts. Clean with plain water. Express colostrum and rub it into the nipples. Wear absorbent pads in the bra if breasts are leaking, but do not allow the wet pad to have prolonged contact with the breast. Leave bra flaps down after nursing. See also Nursing Care Plan 22-2 and Mothers Want to Know: Solutions to Common Breastfeeding Problems.

5. Refer to Mothers Want to Know: Is My Baby Getting Enough Milk?

Home Care of the Infant

Learning Activities

1. Match each term with its definition (a-h).

_____ Babbling

a. Determining whether there is a serious problem that needs follow-up

_____ Colic

b. Cradle cap

_____ Cooing

c. Prickly heat rash

_____ Extrusion reflex

d. Irritable crying for no obvious reason in a healthy infant

_____ Miliaria

e. Using the tongue to push out anything that touches it

_____ Seborrheic dermatitis

f. Vowel sounds made by the infant

_____ Sudden infant death syndrome (SIDS)

g. Consonant sounds made by the infant

_____ Triage

h. Abrupt and unexplained death of an apparently healthy infant

2. Compare advantages and disadvantages of each type of post-discharge follow-up for mothers and infants.

Follow-up	Advantages	Disadvantages
Home visits		
Outpatient visits		
Telephone counseling		

3. What teaching should you give prospective parents about choosing and using an infant car seat for their newborn?
   a. Use of the harness

   b. Direction the seat should face

   c. Safest placement

   d. Use of seat belt with car seat

   e. Use in cars with air bags

4. Suggest at least five things a parent can do for a crying infant who is dry and fed.

a.

b.

c.

d.

e.

5. What should the nurse teach parents about shaken baby syndrome?

6. What should parents be taught about safety when the infant sleeps?

7. How can flattening of the back of the head be prevented?

8. List basic teaching for these parent concerns.
  a. Stools

  b. Smoking around infant

  c. Trimming nails

  d. Pacifiers

9. List expected and abnormal signs associated with teething.
  a. Expected

  b. Abnormal

10. List three aids for diaper rash.

11. Distinguish between spitting up and vomiting.
  a. Spitting up

  b. Vomiting

12. How would you answer a mother who wants to start feeding her 2-month-old infant rice cereal?

13. Approximately when should parents expect each developmental milestone?
   a. Head control

   b. Social smile

   c. Cooing

14. What are the purposes of well-baby check-ups?

15. When should parents seek immediate medical care for their infant?

16. What precautions can parents take to reduce the risk of sudden infant death syndrome?

Check Yourself

1. If a car is equipped with air bags, the newborn's safety seat should always be positioned
   a. Forward-facing in the back seat
   b. Forward-facing in the front seat
   c. Rear-facing in the back seat
   d. Rear-facing in the front seat

2. Parents of a 6-week-old infant are afraid to pick him up if he cries because they do not want to spoil him. The appropriate teaching is that
   a. Infants this young cannot be spoiled by holding in response to crying
   b. They should not worry about crying if he has recently fed well
   c. Holding the infant for no more than 15 minutes at a time usually avoids spoiling
   d. Not holding him will reduce the stimulation that often causes crying

3. At a home visit 3 days after birth, the nurse notes that the infant is swaddled tightly and the room is very warm. Appropriate parent teaching is that
   a. Cold stress will be prevented if the parents continue to dress their baby warmly
   b. The infant can be dressed as they would dress, with the addition of a receiving blanket
   c. Swaddling the infant tightly in a warm room can decrease the severity of colic
   d. Adding a hat and loosening the blankets would be more appropriate dress

4. The best way to cure miliaria is to
   a. Apply cream with a zinc oxide base
   b. Clean the area with mild soap and water
   c. Change the formula to a soy-based one
   d. Take measures to cool the infant

5. A mother is discussing concerns about her 3-month-old infant with the nurse. "She used to nurse for at least 30 minutes each time, but now she seems to finish in 15 to 20 minutes. Do you think I have enough milk for her now?" Today's well-baby check was normal. The nurse's best response is that
   a. The mother should begin weighing her baby before and after each breastfeeding session
   b. Relaxation tapes might help mother and baby relax to encourage longer nursing
   c. Her baby has learned how to nurse more effectively and gets more milk in less time
   d. She should awaken her baby approximately 30 minutes after a feeding and try nursing her again

Developing Insight

1. Find out about laws regarding infant and child safety seats and seat belt use in your state. What is done in your birth facility if parents do not have an infant safety seat at the time of discharge?

2. Does your birth facility have any provisions for routine follow-up for mothers and infants after discharge? Is it available for both well and high-risk infants?

3. How would you teach parents about the importance of immunizations for their infant and child? How should you respond if the parents say the child does not need immunizations because he or she is never taken to daycare centers?

4. Go through your home and identify what changes would be necessary to make it safe for an infant learning to crawl. Use this in teaching parents to anticipate changes that they will have to make in their homes.

ANSWERS TO SELECTED QUESTIONS

Learning Activities

1. g, d, f, e, c, b, h, a
2. Refer to text, pp. 559-562, to complete this exercise.
3. (a) The harness should be easy to fasten with shoulder straps at or just below the shoulder level; restraint clip should be at mid-chest level. (b) The seat for a newborn should face the rear of the vehicle. (c) The safest place is in the center of the back seat. (d) Secure the car seat with the automobile seat belt in the correct area. (e) Do not place car seat in front passenger seat especially if the car has an air bag.
4. See "Parents Want to Know: Methods to Relieve Crying in Infants."
5. When someone shakes a baby, hemorrhage of the brain, fractures, and spinal cord or eye injury can result. Parents should never shake an infant and should seek help if they feel angry enough to do this.
6. Position the infant on the back, not in a prone position. Do not place pillows or soft stuffed toys in the crib. The infant should not sleep with another person or on a soft surface.
7. Placing the infant on the abdomen when awake and supervised and supine at alternating ends of the crib for sleep will help prevent flattening of the head.
8. (a) Formula-fed infants usually pass one stool each day; breastfed infants may have one after each feeding or, when they are older, every 2 or 3 days. Stools should not be hard and dry (constipated) nor should they be watery or leave a water ring on the diaper (diarrhea). Straining and redness in the face when passing stools are normal. (b) There should be no smoking inside the home or near the infant. Infants exposed to smoke have more respiratory infections and a higher incidence of SIDS. (c) Cut nails straight across with a clipper or blunt-ended trimmer, then smooth with an emery board. They should not be cut too short. Cutting them while the infant sleeps may be easier. (d) Discard any pacifier that is cracked, torn, sticky, or pulled away from its shield. Replace pacifiers every 1 to 2 months. Have several clean and ready to use. Never put a pacifier on a string around the neck, but clip it to clothing with a short band. Malocclusion is not a risk unless sucking continues beyond the time the secondary teeth appear.
9. (a) Excessive salivation, biting, irritability, slight fever, reduced appetite, red or swollen gums, rash around the mouth, night wakening; (b) high fever, other signs of illness
10. Any of these remedies may be used: change diapers as soon as possible when wet or soiled; wash the area gently with soap and water; expose the area to air; apply a thin layer of petrolatum or zinc oxide cream.
11. (a) In spitting up, a small amount of milk is lost with the burp; it is not forcefully expelled. (b) Vomiting involves a large amount of milk, vomited with force. If it continues, the parents should report it to the health care provider.
12. Use the following facts in formulating your answer: Early feeding of solids can increase allergies and replaces milk, which is easily digested, with a food that is not taken or digested well. The extrusion reflex makes feeding of solids difficult until the age of 4 to 6 months. Early feeding may lead to obesity and will not help the infant sleep through the night.
13. (a) 3 months; (b) 1 to 3 months; (c) 1 to 4 months
14. Well-baby check-ups assess growth and development, answer parent questions, identify abnormalities, and allow infants to receive immunizations.
15. If signs of dyspnea occur (sustained respiratory rate greater than 60 breaths per minute [bpm] or less than 30 bpm, retractions, cyanosis, or extreme pallor) or the infant is hard to arouse, parents should see their pediatrician or visit an emergency department. Sudden respiratory distress in a well infant may indicate aspiration, and parents should summon paramedics.
16. Avoid having the infant sleep in a prone position, overheating the infant, or letting the infant sleep with another person; provide a firm sleeping surface; allow no loose blankets, pillows, or stuffed toys in the infant's bed; avoid smoking.

Check Yourself

1, c; 2, a; 3, b; 4, d; 5, c

The Childbearing Family with Special Needs

Learning Activities

1. Match each term with its definition (a-e).

_____ Crack   a. Interest centered on self rather than on others

_____ Egocentrism   b. Long-acting drug to substitute for heroin or morphine

_____ Honeymoon phase   c. Highly addictive form of cocaine

_____ Methadone   d. Drugs such as morphine, heroin, methadone, meperidine

_____ Opiates   e. Time after a battering incident when the partner is very solicitous of the woman

2. Explain how pregnancy affects the adolescent's
   a. Development of independence

   b. Education

   c. Employment opportunities

3. What pregnancy risks are higher for adolescents than for adults?

4. What problems are more likely for the children of an adolescent mother?

5. What can be done to increase the adolescent's likelihood to come for regular prenatal care?

6. List complications the mature pregnant woman is more likely to encounter.
  a. Genetic

  b. Preexisting disorders

  c. Obstetric complications

7. What problems is the mature mother likely to encounter in terms of
  a. Fatigue

  b. Support of friends or family

8. Why do substances taken by the mother tend to have a more pronounced effect on her fetus than on her?

9. Complete the following chart related to fetal and neonatal effects of maternal substance use.

	Fetal Effects	*Neonatal Effects*
Tobacco		
Alcohol		
Marijuana		
Cocaine		
Amphetamines and methamphetamines		
Opioids		
Sedatives (barbiturates)		
Selective serotonin reuptake inhibitors		

10. Why might the nurse suspect a woman may have used cocaine if she is admitted in preterm labor and having intense contractions?

11. List antepartal signs associated with drug abuse.
   a. Behaviors

   b. Physical appearance

   c. Medical history

   d. Obstetric history

   e. Emotional reaction to pregnancy

12. What signs might the woman have during the intrapartum period if she has recently ingested these drugs?
   a. Cocaine

   b. Heroin

13. What special concerns might parents have if the infant has facial or genital anomalies?

14. Why is grief an essential aspect of attachment to an infant with an anomaly?

15. Why is it important that both fathers and mothers be supported in the grief aspects of having a baby with an anomaly or of perinatal loss?

16. Describe the risks to an abused pregnant woman and her fetus.
    a. Woman

    b. Fetus

17. Describe each phase of the violence cycle.
    a.

    b.

    c.

18. Every woman should be screened for abuse when receiving health care. What questions should be asked to identify intimate partner violence?

Check Yourself

1. The best way for the nurse to evaluate the quality of a pregnant adolescent's diet is to
   a. Ask her, in a nonthreatening manner, how well she eats
   b. Assume it is inadequate and give her advice
   c. Ask her to describe what she ate the previous day
   d. Have her record everything she eats for 1 week

2. In providing teaching for the pregnant adolescent the nurse should
   a. Provide plenty of written material for her to study at home
   b. Not expect her to be interested in learning about pregnancy
   c. Teach her in small groups along with other pregnant teens
   d. Avoid audiovisual aids because she will not respond to them

3. Correct advice for women who ask about using alcohol during pregnancy is that it is
  a. Safest if taken only during the last trimester
  b. Best to avoid alcohol during the first 12 weeks
  c. Unknown if there is any fetal harm from alcohol use
  d. Important to avoid alcohol throughout pregnancy

4. A woman who has been taking methadone during her pregnancy asks for pain medicine during labor. The nurse should
  a. Call the physician to obtain an order for a safe pain medication
  b. Realize that her methadone is enough to control the pain of labor
  c. Expect the physician to order butorphanol (Stadol) for her pain
  d. Expect that she will need only a very small dose of medication

5. When first presenting an infant with an anomaly to parents, the nurse should
  a. Have the physician initially discuss the causes of the anomaly, if known
  b. Point out normal aspects of the infant, as well as showing them the anomaly
  c. Wait until the mother has had time to recuperate from the stress of labor
  d. Limit their time with the infant the first time they see him or her

6. A woman who had a stillborn infant at 37 weeks of gestation angrily asks the nurse why her physician didn't "take the baby early." The nurse should understand that the mother's behavior
  a. Is unusual when stillbirth occurs at this late gestation
  b. Suggests discord between the woman and her partner
  c. Should be expected as part of the normal grieving process
  d. Reflects intense guilt about her own self-care in pregnancy

7. When preparing a memory packet for parents after a fetal demise the nurse will include
  a. The infant's footprints, a lock of hair
  b. A copy of the delivery records
  c. A blood sample for DNA testing
  d. Explanation of the cause of the demise

8. In caring for a woman who has experienced a perinatal loss the nurse should
  a. Allow her to be alone as much as possible to cope with her loss
  b. Acknowledge the loss and ask how the nurse can be of help
  c. Provide nursing care without mentioning the loss
  d. Help her explore how she might prevent another loss

9. A woman shows injuries that may have been caused by abuse. Which of the following should the nurse do first?
  a. Call the police and help the woman complete a report.
  b. Confront the woman and her partner with her suspicions.
  c. Tell the woman she should leave her partner immediately.
  d. Find a way to talk with the woman away from her partner.

10. The main goal in caring for victims of intimate partner abuse is to
  a. Emphasize that they have the right not to be hurt
  b. Help them better identify their role in the family
  c. Encourage them to ask their partners about counseling
  d. Limit their ability to return to the abusive partner

11. What are the advantages of childbirth in the mature woman over the young woman?
  a. The woman will have more common sense than a younger mother.
  b. She will have planned the timing of the pregnancy carefully.
  c. She will love her infant more than a younger mother.
  d. She is more likely to be financially secure and have more self-confidence.

Developing Insight

1. If you care for a teenage mother, discuss the involvement of the infant's father and the grandmother in infant care. What are the future plans of the young mother (and father, if involved)? Are their plans realistic? Why or why not? Did the girl attend school during her pregnancy and what are her future plans for education?

2. What programs are available in your community for teenage parents, both during pregnancy and after they give birth?

3. What does your state require if either the mother or the infant shows evidence of drug abuse in toxicology screens?

4. Talk with your hospital's emergency department personnel about their experiences with victims of intimate partner abuse. Do they note any differences in abuse when a woman is pregnant?

ANSWERS TO SELECTED QUESTIONS

Learning Activities

1. c, a, e, b, d

2. (a) Development of independence from parents is interrupted; the teenage girl usually becomes more dependent on them financially and emotionally, rather than becoming more independent. (b) Education is often interrupted and may never be completed, but some adolescents become motivated to change and become more goal-directed. (c) Reliance on the welfare system is more likely because of incomplete education and limited job skills.

3. Preeclampsia, anemia, cephalopelvic disproportion, preterm labor and birth, perinatal mortality, low-birth-weight infants, depression, abusive relationship, and sexually transmitted diseases (STDs)

4. Children of teen mothers are more likely to have impaired intellectual functioning and poor school adjustment. In addition, they tend to repeat the cycle and become teenage parents themselves.

5. Adolescents are more likely to seek regular prenatal care if they go to caregivers who are located in convenient locations and who have after-school appointments and if attitudes of staff are friendly and accepting of their special needs.

6. (a) Higher incidence of chromosome abnormalities such as Down syndrome. (b) Increased likelihood of underlying chronic conditions that complicate pregnancy, such as diabetes, hypertension, and myomas. (c) Higher incidence of spontaneous abortion, preeclampsia, gestational diabetes, placenta previa, multifetal gestation, preterm labor and birth, prolonged labor, dystocia, cesarean birth, and fetal demise.

7. (a) She may have less energy to cope with the demands of an infant plus the day-to-day activities of living. (b) She may have less peer and family support because most other women her age have teenagers or young adults and family members may not be available.

8. Most substances taken by the mother cross the placenta and enter the fetal circulation. The fetus cannot metabolize the substance as quickly, so the substance lingers for a prolonged time in the fetal body.

9. Refer to text, Table 24-2, to complete this exercise.

10. Cocaine directly stimulates uterine contractions. Abruptio placentae, premature rupture of the membranes, preeclampsia, fetal hypoxia, meconium staining, and need for resuscitation at birth are more likely to occur, and the nurse should be prepared for these possibilities, as well as for complications in the newborn.

11. (a) Late prenatal care, failing to keep appointments, not following recommendations, defensive or hostile behavior. (b) Poor grooming, inadequate weight gain, weight gain pattern that does not conform to that expected for the gestational age, fresh needle punctures, signs of cellulitis or thrombosed veins. (c) Depression, seizures, hepatitis, pneumonia, cellulitis, STDs, hypertension, suicide attempts, insomnia, panic attacks, exhaustion, heart palpitations. (d) Spontaneous abortions, premature births, abruptio placentae, stillbirths. (e) Anger or apathy toward pregnancy, especially late in the pregnancy.

12. (a) Profuse sweating, hypertension, irregular respirations, lethargic response to labor, lack of interest in interventions, dilated pupils, increased body temperature, sudden onset of severely painful contractions, anger, emotional lability and paranoia, fetal tachycardia or bradycardia, late decelerations, and fetal hyperactivity. (b) Withdrawal symptoms such as yawning, diaphoresis, rhinorrhea, restlessness, excessive tearing, nausea, vomiting, abdominal cramping.

13. Facial abnormalities cause parental concerns about how others will accept their child, because the defect is obvious. Genital defects cause ambiguity and anxiety about the child's identity—is the baby a boy or a girl? How should the baby be dressed? What name should be given?

14. Parents must grieve for the loss of the expected normal child before they can detach from this fantasy and move on to accepting the child they have.

15. The father, as well as the mother, must be assisted to deal with the shock and sadness, rather than all attention being focused on the mother's grief. Only when the father has help to cope with his emotions can he support his partner and explain the loss to the couple's family and friends.

16. (a) Multiple injury sites, especially of the abdomen, face, and breasts; late entry into prenatal care; vaginal bleeding, severe nausea and vomiting, kidney or urinary tract infections, low maternal weight gain, anemia; more likely to use substances. (b) Spontaneous abortion, prematurity, abruptio placentae, low birth-weight, fetal death.

17. (a) *Tension-building*, when threats and angry behaviors escalate; increased use of alcohol and drugs; the woman tries to avoid or placate her abuser. (b) *Battering*, with hitting, burning, beating, or raping the woman. The woman often simply endures the abuse. (c) *Honeymoon phase*, when the abuser is overly solicitous and tries to make up with his partner. He often insists on having intercourse to prove that she forgives him. The woman wants to believe that he will never abuse her again.

18. Any questioning should be done when the woman is alone to avoid repercussions to her later from her abuser. Tell the woman that all women are asked the

same questions. Include inquires about being hit, slapped, forced to have sex, or otherwise hurt by someone within the last year; whether it has happened during the pregnancy; and whether she is afraid of anyone. Other questions will follow depending on the woman's answers.

Check Yourself

1, c; 2, c; 3, d; 4, a; 5, b; 6, c; 7, a; 8, b; 9, d; 10, a; 11, d

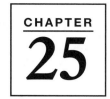

Complications of Pregnancy

Learning Activities

1. Match each term with its definition (a-h).

_____ Cerclage

a. The embryo or fetus, plus the placenta and membranes

_____ Ectopic pregnancy

b. Material that absorbs water and expands to dilate the cervix

_____ HELLP

c. Erythrocyte fragmentation, hyperbilirubinemia, and thrombocytopenia that may occur in preeclampsia

_____ K-B test

d. Implantation of the fertilized ovum outside the uterine cavity

_____ Kernicterus

e. Encircling the cervix with sutures

_____ *Laminaria*

f. Bilirubin accumulation within the brain that may cause damage

_____ Maceration

g. Degeneration of a fetus retained in the uterus after its death

_____ Products of conception

h. Identifying presence of fetal erythrocytes into maternal circulation

2. Define *spontaneous abortion*. What is another term for this occurrence?

3. Complete the following table on types of spontaneous abortions.

	Clinical Manifestations	*Therapeutic Management*
Threatened		
Inevitable		
Incomplete		
Complete		
Missed		
Recurrent		

4. Describe altered laboratory studies that may be seen in disseminated intravascular coagulopathy (DIC).
  a. Fibrinogen

  b. Platelets

  c. Prothrombin time (PT)

  d. Activated partial thromboplastin time (aPTT)

  e. D-dimer

5. Write a simply worded response that you might use if a woman expresses the feeling that she did something to cause her spontaneous abortion. Have you or someone close experienced a loss of early pregnancy? List any specific risk factors if you have cared for a woman who has had a spontaneous abortion.

6. What is the possible significance of sudden pain in the area of the scapula during early pregnancy? What factors increase a woman's risk of an ectopic pregnancy?

7. What teaching is needed for the woman having methotrexate therapy for an early ectopic pregnancy?

8. List the typical signs and symptoms of gestational trophoblastic disease. What is another name for this complication?

9. What is the relationship between gestational trophoblastic disease and cancer? What precautions related to cancer detection are taken before and after evacuation of the abnormal tissue?

10. List foods that should be emphasized for a woman who experienced a bleeding complication of pregnancy (at any gestation). How would you explain, simply, the need for these foods? What changes would you make to your suggestions if the woman is vegetarian or from a group with specific diet preferences or guidelines?

11. Complete the following chart to compare placenta previa with abruptio placentae.

	Placenta Previa	*Abruptio Placentae*
Placenta location		
Character of bleeding		
Presence of pain		
Uterine activity		
Diagnosis		

12. List nursing teaching associated with home care when a woman has placenta previa.

13. What is the relationship between cocaine use and abruptio placentae?

14. Why is the amount of external bleeding in abruptio placentae not a reliable indicator of the true amount of blood loss?

15. List early and late signs of hypovolemic shock.
   a. Early

   b. Late

16. List nursing measures and their rationales to promote maternal and fetal oxygenation if hemorrhage occurs or is suspected at 37 weeks of gestation.

17. Describe how generalized vasospasm of preeclampsia affects each organ and how these effects are manifested.
  a. Kidneys

  b. Liver

  c. Brain

  d. Lungs

  e. Placenta

18. What are the classic signs of preeclampsia? What nonspecific sign may occur?

19. What is the significance of epigastric pain in a woman with preeclampsia?

20. List signs of magnesium toxicity. When is toxicity more likely to occur?

21. What is the antidote for magnesium toxicity?

22. What features distinguish chronic hypertension from hypertension of pregnancy? Can the two types occur at the same time?

23. What conditions are necessary for a woman to receive Rho(D) immune globulin? What does each mean?
   a. Rh factor of the woman

   b. Rh factor of the fetus or newborn

   c. Indirect Coombs' test (woman)

   d. Direct Coombs' test (newborn)

24. How can ABO incompatibility occur?

Check Yourself

1. Choose the primary distinction between threatened and inevitable abortion.
   a. Presence of cramping
   b. Rupture of membranes
   c. Vaginal bleeding
   d. Pelvic pressure

2. A woman is admitted to the emergency department with a possible ectopic pregnancy. Choose the sign or symptom that should be immediately reported to her physician.
   a. Low level of beta-hCG (human chorionic gonadotropin)
   b. Hemoglobin of 11.5 g/dL; hematocrit of 34%
   c. Light vaginal bleeding
   d. Pulse rises from 78 to 112 beats per minute (bpm)

3. When caring for a woman who has had a hydatidiform mole evacuated, the clinic nurse's priority intervention is to
   a. Reinforce the need to delay a new pregnancy for 1 year
   b. Ask the woman whether she has any cramping or bleeding
   c. Observe return of her blood pressure to normal
   d. Palpate the uterus for return to its normal size

4. The woman who is receiving methotrexate for an ectopic pregnancy should be cautioned to avoid
   a. Driving or operating machinery
   b. Eating raw vegetables or fruits
   c. Using latex condoms for intercourse
   d. Taking vitamins with folic acid

5. A woman who is 34 weeks pregnant is admitted with contractions every 2 minutes, lasting 60 seconds, and a high uterine resting tone. She says she had some vaginal bleeding at home, and there is a small amount of blood on her perineal pad. The priority action of the nurse is to
   a. Establish whether she is in labor by performing a vaginal examination
   b. Ask her whether she has had recent intercourse or a vaginal examination
   c. Evaluate the maternal and fetal circulation and oxygenation
   d. Determine whether this is the first episode of pain she has had

6. Nursing teaching for the woman who has hyperemesis gravidarum should include which of the following?
   a. Adding favorite seasonings to foods while cooking
   b. Eating simple foods such as breads and fruits
   c. Lying down on the right side after eating
   d. Eating creamed soup with every meal

7. The nurse makes the following assessments of a woman who is receiving intravenous magnesium sulfate: fetal heart rate (FHR), 148 to 158 bpm; pulse, 88 bpm; respirations, 9 breaths per minute; blood pressure, 158/96 mm Hg. The woman is drowsy. The priority nursing action is to
   a. Increase the rate of the magnesium infusion
   b. Maintain the magnesium infusion at the current rate
   c. Slow the rate of the magnesium infusion
   d. Stop the magnesium infusion

8. When providing intrapartum care for the woman with severe preeclampsia, priority nursing care is to
   a. Maintain the ordered rate of anticonvulsant medications
   b. Promote placental blood flow and prevent maternal injury
   c. Give intravenous fluids and observe urine output
   d. Reduce maternal blood pressure to the prepregnancy level

9. Clonus indicates which of the following?
   a. Central nervous system is very irritable.
   b. Renal blood flow is severely reduced.
   c. Lungs are filling with interstitial fluid.
   d. Muscles of the foot are inflamed.

10. The feature that distinguishes preeclampsia from eclampsia is the
    a. Amount of blood pressure elevation
    b. Edema of the face and fingers
    c. Presence of 4+ proteinuria
    d. Onset of one or more seizures

11. Which woman should receive Rho(D) immune globulin after birth?
    a. Rh-negative mother; Rh-positive infant; positive direct Coombs' test
    b. Rh-positive mother; Rh-negative infant; negative direct Coombs' test
    c. Rh-negative mother; Rh-positive infant; negative direct Coombs' test
    d. Rh-positive mother; Rh-positive infant; positive direct Coombs' test

Developing Insight

1. Ask staff nurses at your clinical facility about their experiences with women who have hyperemesis gravidarum. Do you detect any preset beliefs about the disorder among the nurses? What is the usual plan of treatment for a woman with hyperemesis who is in the first trimester?

2. Discuss factors you encounter in your clinical facility that may contribute to a woman's hypertension. If she had no or late prenatal care, would the physician be able to determine whether her hypertension was caused by preeclampsia or was chronic hypertension? Why?

Case Study

Patricia is a 17-year-old gravida 1, para 0 at 34 weeks of gestation, who is visiting her physician for a routine prenatal visit. When weighing Patricia, the nurse finds that she has gained 6 lb in the past 2 weeks.

1. What is the main objective after this initial assessment?

2. What is the most important question or problem that must be solved during Patricia's prenatal visit?

3. What are the nurse's priority assessments? Why?

The nurse obtains a clean-catch urine specimen from Patricia and takes her vital signs (temperature, 37° C [98.6° F]; pulse, 82 bpm; respirations, 20 breaths per minute; blood pressure, 146/90 mm Hg); the FHR is 144 to 150 bpm. Deep tendon reflexes are normal (2+), and no clonus is present.

4. What testing would you expect to be performed on the urine specimen? Why?

5. What information might the nurse need from previous prenatal visits and why?

6. What questions should the nurse ask Patricia while assessing her?

Patricia's physician diagnoses mild preeclampsia and will initially manage Patricia at home.

7. What findings would lead the physician to the diagnosis of mild preeclampsia?

8. Why do you think the physician is recommending home management at this time?

9. What teaching is essential regarding Patricia's home care? Do you think it is important to include a family member in teaching? Discuss reasons for including others in Patricia's teaching with one or more classmates and list the group's reasons here.

ANSWERS TO SELECTED QUESTIONS

Learning Activities

1. e, d, c, h, f, b, g, a
2. Termination of a pregnancy without action taken by the woman or any other person. *Miscarriage* is usually used by laypeople but is becoming more common in usage by professionals.
3. Refer to text, pp. 616-618, to complete this exercise.
4. (a) Fibrinogen decreased; (b) platelets decreased; (c) prothrombin time prolonged; (d) activated partial thromboplastin time prolonged; (e) D-dimer positive, confirming fibrin split products
5. Refer to text, p. 618, to formulate your explanation. If desired, incorporate personal experiences of early pregnancy loss into your explanation.
6. Abrupt onset of shoulder pain may occur with a ruptured ectopic pregnancy, because blood accumulated in the abdomen irritates the phrenic nerve. Refer to Box 25-1, p. 619, to list risk factors.
7. Explain the side effects, such as nausea and vomiting. Teach the woman to refrain from drinking alcohol, ingesting vitamins with folic acid, or having sexual intercourse until human chorionic gonadotropin (hCG) is not detectable in the serum (usually 2 to 4 weeks). Keeping follow-up appointments should also be emphasized.
8. Elevated hCG; vaginal bleeding that varies in amount and color; uterine enlargement greater than expected for the gestation; undetectable fetal heart activity or ultrasound pattern with characteristic vesicles; excessive nausea and vomiting; early onset of preeclampsia. Hydatidiform mole is another name for gestational trophoblastic disease.
9. Most tissue in gestational trophoblastic disease is benign, but choriocarcinoma is a possibility. Before the abnormal tissue is evacuated, the woman will be evaluated for metastatic disease. Serum hCG will be evaluated every 1 to 2 weeks until normal levels are attained and then repeated every 1 to 2 months for 1 year. Pregnancy must be avoided during this period.
10. Foods high in iron should be emphasized to aid in restoring hemoglobin levels and to aid in the body's defense against infection. These include liver, red meat, spinach, egg yolks, carrots, and raisins. Foods high in vitamin C may help iron to be utilized more effectively. Use the information in Chapter 9 to formulate your explanation.
11. Refer to text, pp. 624-627, to complete this chart.
12. The woman and her family should be taught to assess the vaginal discharge, fetal movement counts, and uterine activity. She should be given guidelines for what to report. Curtailment of sexual intercourse and return physician visits should be discussed, as well. Developing a plan of care suitable for the individual family improves the likelihood of safe home management and that emergency care will be started immediately if the need arises.
13. Cocaine is a vasoconstrictor, including constriction of the uterine endometrial arteries, which may lead to premature placental separation.
14. Much or all of the blood may be trapped by the placenta, which may remain attached at the edges.
15. (a) Tachycardia, diminished peripheral pulses, normal or slightly decreased blood pressure, tachypnea, pallor and coolness of the skin and mucous membranes. (b) Falling blood pressure, pallor, skin that is cold and clammy, urine output less than 30 mL/hr, restlessness, agitation, decreased mentation
16. (In any order) Lateral positioning with the head flat to increase cardiac return and enhance circulation to the placenta and vital organs; limited maternal movement to reduce demand for oxygen; providing explanations, reassurance, and emotional support to reduce anxiety that would increase maternal demand for oxygen
17. (a) Reduced blood flow causes a reduced glomerular filtration rate, which causes a rise in blood urea nitrogen (BUN), creatinine, and uric acid. Glomerular damage caused by reduced perfusion allows protein to leak across the glomerular membrane, resulting in interstitial fluid accumulation, hypovolemia, and increased blood viscosity and hematocrit (hemoconcentration). Angiotensin II and aldosterone are secreted in response to hypovolemia, further increasing the blood pressure. (b) Reduced perfusion decreases liver function. Hepatic edema and subcapsular hemorrhage may occur. Serum may have elevated liver enzymes. (c) Vasoconstriction leads to pressure-induced rupture of small capillaries, resulting in small cerebral hemorrhages. Symptoms such as headache and visual disturbances may result. (d) Reduced oncotic pressure can result in pulmonary edema. (e) Reduced perfusion can cause infarctions or abruptio placentae. The risk of disseminated intravascular coagulopathy is also higher. The fetus may have growth restriction and persistent hypoxemia, resulting in fetal acidosis, mental retardation, or death.
18. Hypertension (systolic blood pressure ≥140 mm Hg or diastolic blood pressure ≥90 mm Hg) and proteinuria. Edema may occur. Expected edema of pregnancy is usually mild and remains in the feet and legs. If edema accompanies other signs of preeclampsia it may be preceded by sudden weight gain and may be above the waist.
19. Epigastric pain occurs with hepatic capsule distention, which often heralds an imminent seizure.
20. Central nervous system depression, possibly resulting in diminished or absent deep tendon reflexes, respiratory

depression, and hypotension. Reduced urinary output can cause magnesium to accumulate to unsafe levels. Toxicity is more likely if serum level is greater than 8 mg/dL.

21. Calcium gluconate
22. Chronic hypertension is present before pregnancy or before 20 weeks of gestation and may occur with hypertension of pregnancy.
23. (a) The woman must have Rh-negative blood because she will not make anti-Rh antibodies if she is Rh-positive. (b) The newborn must have Rh-positive blood because Rh-negative blood cannot induce development of anti-Rh antibodies in the Rh-negative woman. (c) Indirect Coombs' test should be negative, indicating that the woman has not made anti-Rh antibodies (become sensitized) to Rh-positive blood during the pregnancy. (d) The direct Coombs' test identifies maternal antibodies in the newborn's blood and should be negative.
24. ABO incompatibility can occur if a type O mother has a fetus that is type A, B, or AB, because these blood types contain an antigen that is not present on type O erythrocytes. Many type O people have developed high levels of antibodies to blood types A, B, or AB, and the antibodies can cross the placenta and damage fetal erythrocytes that are one of these types. The effects are usually less severe than Rh incompatibility.

Check Yourself

1, b; 2, d; 3, a; 4, d; 5, c; 6, b; 7, d; 8, b; 9, a; 10, d; 11, c

Case Study

1. The main objective of the nurse's assessment is to identify why Patricia had a sudden excessive weight gain. Preeclampsia is a likely suspect, but the nurse must assess for other possible causes, such as a substantially increased food intake or sudden decrease in activity. Excessive salt intake is another possibility.

2. The staff must determine whether Patricia's weight gain is the result of preeclampsia and take steps to treat it.
3. The nurse should assess for other signs and symptoms because preeclampsia is a serious complication of pregnancy: hypertension and elevated urine protein, often accompanied by severe edema; epigastric pain; visual disturbances such as spots or blurring; severe and unrelenting headache; dyspnea.
4. A dipstick test for proteinuria would be performed to identify excessive levels of protein in the urine. Reduced kidney perfusion causes glomerular damage, causing loss of protein in the urine. Testing for glucose and ketones or other tests might be performed, although these do not directly relate to preeclampsia.
5. The nurse needs Patricia's past pattern of weight gain and her previous vital signs to evaluate today's information more accurately.
6. The nurse should ask Patricia whether her rings are tighter than usual (finger edema), whether she sees spots in front of her eyes or has blurring of vision or whether she has had severe headaches (cerebral edema), whether she has upper abdominal pain or nausea (distended liver capsule), and whether she has difficulty in breathing (pulmonary edema).
7. Refer to Table 25-2, p. 636, to complete this question.
8. Patricia's preeclampsia is mild, and the fetal signs are favorable. Because the fetus is at 34 weeks of gestation, delay of birth would be good unless Patricia's preeclampsia worsens. In that case, poor placental perfusion is likely to cause the fetus more problems—including possible fetal demise—than preterm delivery.
9. Teaching involves activity restrictions, including how to achieve them; assessment of fetal activity; maternal blood pressure; weight; and urine protein. The woman and family must be taught what signs and symptoms to report and when to return for fetal surveillance studies and frequent prenatal visits. List reasons that you and classmates identify for including family or significant others in Patricia's teaching.

Concurrent Disorders during Pregnancy

Learning Activities

1. Match each term with its definition (a-f).

_____ Anemia   a. Delayed or difficult birth of the fetal shoulders

_____ Ketosis   b. Period of major fetal organ development

_____ Organogenesis   c. Hemoglobin concentration lower than 10.5 to 11.0 g/dl

_____ Pica   d. Development of antibodies in response to infection or immunization

_____ Seroconversion
                                      e. May be associated with excess acid in blood

_____ Shoulder dystocia
                                      f. Consumption of nonfood substances

2. List and explain the four classic signs of diabetes in the type that requires insulin.

a.

b.

c.

d.

3. How does diabetes alter food metabolism during pregnancy?
a. Early pregnancy

b. Late pregnancy

4. Why is maintenance of a normal blood glucose level before and during early pregnancy particularly important?

5. What are the effects of maternal vascular involvement on the fetus/newborn of a diabetic mother?

6. Do insulin needs increase, decrease, or remain stable during the following times? Why?
a. First trimester

b. Second and third trimesters

c. Labor

d. Postpartum

7. When would a physician want a pregnant woman to have an oral glucose tolerance test (OGTT)?

8. What steps minimize insulin leakage from an injection site?

9. Why is it recommended that a woman who has hypoglycemia avoid sucrose or unrefined sugar, such as candy to raise her glucose level to normal?

10. List early signs and symptoms of congestive heart failure.

11. Janet is a 26-year-old woman who is 30 weeks pregnant with her first baby. She has rheumatic heart disease. She had to stop working at her desk job at 20 weeks of pregnancy because of persistent fatigue. She has no problems when sitting quietly, but tasks such as making her bed or gathering laundry to wash cause her to have slight chest pain and a rapid heartbeat. She complains that she always feels tired. What class of heart disease do her symptoms suggest? Why?

12. What anticoagulant is recommended if needed during pregnancy? Why?

13. Why are labor and the immediate postpartum period especially dangerous for a woman who has heart disease?

14. A woman who is 32 weeks pregnant and has class II heart disease visits the antepartum clinic for a routine visit. You find that she has gained 7 lb since her visit 1 week ago. Is her weight gain normal for gestation? What possibilities should you consider?

15. Why is it important to take adequate folic acid before and during pregnancy?

16. Why does maternal sickle cell crisis make fetal death more likely?

17. Describe the signs and symptoms of sickle cell crisis.

18. List pregnancy-associated risks for the woman who has systemic lupus erythematosus and her fetus/neonate.

19. Why is drug management of the woman who has a seizure disorder such as epilepsy difficult during pregnancy?

20. Describe the four stages in the course of human immunodeficiency virus (HIV) infection. If you have cared for anyone with HIV, describe his or her stage and the signs and symptoms the person displayed.
   a.

   b.

   c.

   d.

21. Complete the following table to learn more about viral infections during pregnancy.

Infection	Maternal Effects	Fetal and Neonatal Effects	Prevention	Treatment
Cytomegalovirus				
Rubella				
Varicella zoster				
Herpesviruses				
Parvovirus B19				
Hepatitis B				

22. At what point is a person said to have acquired immunodeficiency syndrome (AIDS)?

23. What drugs are available to benefit people infected with HIV? Which one is recommended for HIV-infected pregnant women to prevent viral transmission to the fetus?

24. What nursing care is appropriate for the HIV-infected pregnant woman? If you have cared for anyone with HIV infection, describe the nursing care and medical management the person needed. Include men and nonpregnant women or children in your description(s).

25. Complete the following table to learn more about nonviral infections during pregnancy.

Infection	Maternal Effects	Fetal and Neonatal Effects	Prevention	Treatment
Toxoplasmosis				
Group B streptococcus				
Tuberculosis				

Check Yourself

1. The test used to screen for gestational diabetes is the
   a. Glycosylated hemoglobin test
   b. Glucose challenge test
   c. Oral glucose tolerance test
   d. Postprandial glucose test

2. The best evaluation for the client's goal of accurate insulin administration is that she will
   a. Repeat the steps taught for insulin injection verbally
   b. Accurately withdraw, mix, and inject insulin
   c. Have normal fasting and postprandial glucose levels
   d. State that she understands the teaching given

3. Rheumatic heart disease is usually preceded by which infection?
   a. Streptococcal pharyngitis
   b. Primary syphilis
   c. Pneumococcal pneumonia
   d. Chlamydial vaginitis

4. The primary fetal risk when the mother has any type of anemia is for
   a. Neonatal anemia
   b. Elevated bilirubin
   c. Limited infection defenses
   d. Reduced oxygen delivery

5. Intrapartum nursing care for a woman who has sickle cell disease focuses on
   a. Maintaining oxygenation and preventing dehydration
   b. Controlling pain and avoiding unnecessary movement
   c. Preventing excess exertion and limiting visitors
   d. Increasing calorie intake and avoiding internal monitoring

6. When caring for a pregnant woman who has antiphospholipid syndrome, the clinic nurse must especially observe for development of
   a. Urinary tract infections
   b. Nausea and vomiting
   c. Elevated blood pressure
   d. Reduced blood glucose

7. Reduction in congenital rubella is best accomplished by
   a. Avoiding contact with young children when infections are prevalent
   b. Taking prophylactic antibiotics during the second half of pregnancy
   c. Testing the rubella titer at the first prenatal visit to determine immunity
   d. Immunizing susceptible women at least 28 days before they become pregnant

8. The pregnant woman who becomes infected with chickenpox should be taught to report promptly
   a. Cough or dyspnea
   b. Severe skin itching
   c. Joint pain
   d. Increased urination

9. Choose the appropriate infant care teaching for a woman who gave birth by cesarean because of active genital herpes.
   a. Do not breastfeed the infant until all lesions are healed.
   b. Thoroughly wash your hands before handling the infant.
   c. Wear a mask when breastfeeding or holding the infant close.
   d. No special precautions are needed when caring for the infant.

10. Correct injection technique for infants of mothers who are known carriers of hepatitis B virus is to
    a. Avoid all intramuscular injections until 1 month of age
    b. Dilute intramuscular injections with added normal saline
    c. Mix all injections the infant will need in a single syringe
    d. Bathe the area where the infant will receive injections

11. For HIV treatment the pregnant woman should be expected to receive
    a. Antibiotics
    b. Protease analogs
    c. Zidovudine
    d. Acyclovir

12. Expected drug treatment for a pregnant woman who has tuberculosis is
    a. Acyclovir and zidovudine
    b. Ampicillin and gentamicin
    c. Cefotaxime, levofloxacin, and vancomycin
    d. Isoniazid, pyrazinamide, and rifampin

Developing Insight

1. Review charts to determine whether clients had a glucose challenge test and their response to it. What follow-up was done if their blood level was 140 mg/dl or higher? Is a different glucose level used at your clinical facility?

2. Calculate your own calorie allowance if you were pregnant based on the formula stated in the text.

3. How are insulin infusions managed in your facility if a pregnant woman cannot eat, such as during labor or surgery?

4. Examine your attitudes toward people with HIV. Are you fearful of them? Did you have to confront this fear before entering nursing school? How do you feel about pregnant women who have HIV? Are your feelings for "innocent" victims, such as infants, different from feelings for those who acquired the infection through unsafe sexual practices or intravenous (IV) drug use?

Case Study

Debra is a 22-year-old gravida 1, para 0, who has had type I (insulin-dependent) diabetes for 6 years. Her last menstrual period was 12 weeks ago.

1. How will Debra's diabetes be affected by her pregnancy?

2. What changes will she most likely need to make in her diabetes management because she is pregnant?

3. What routine assessments will be made at each prenatal visit?

4. What additional tests will Debra need as her pregnancy progresses?

5. How may Debra's fetus be affected by her diabetes?

6. What nursing management during labor should be expected?

7. What newborn problems should the nurse anticipate?

8. What added care will Debra's infant need?

ANSWERS TO SELECTED QUESTIONS

Learning Activities

1. c, e, b, f, d, a

2. (In any order) (a) Polydipsia (excess thirst as the body attempts to dilute glucose load with fluid drawn from intracellular space); (b) polyuria (excess urine output as the body uses osmotic diuresis to excrete excess glucose); (c) polyphagia (excess appetite as the body attempts to metabolize food to provide glucose for normal cell metabolism); (d) weight loss (cell starvation despite large food intake)

3. (a) Early pregnancy: Little change in maternal metabolic rate and energy need; increasing insulin release in response to serum glucose, often leading to hypoglycemia; nausea and vomiting increase likelihood of hypoglycemia; glucose and insulin availability favors fat storage to prepare for fetal energy use during second trimester. (b) Late pregnancy: Rise in placental hormones (estrogen, progesterone, human placental lactogen) creates insulin resistance, allowing abundant glucose supply to be available to fetus. The same hormones can create hyperglycemia in the mother if her pancreas cannot respond with increased insulin to metabolize increased glucose.

4. Hypoglycemia and hyperglycemia are associated with more spontaneous abortions, congenital malformations, hypertension, urinary tract infections, and a greater tendency toward ketoacidosis. Fetal complications can include hydramnios, premature rupture of the membranes, intrauterine growth restriction, and abnormal fetal size. Neonatal effects include hypoglycemia, hypocalcemia, hyperbilirubinemia, and respiratory distress syndrome.

5. With no vascular impairment, hyperglycemia can lead to macrosomia if the mother's glucose levels remain high or poorly controlled. Vascular impairment limits glucose and oxygen transport to the fetus and can result in intrauterine growth restriction.

6. (a) First trimester: Insulin needs decrease because of reduced maternal food intake and uptake of glucose by embryo/fetus. (b) Second and third trimesters: Needs increase because of maternal insulin resistance and greater food intake. (c) Labor: Needs usually decrease because of exertion and reduced food intake. (d) Postpartum: Needs decrease because of loss of hormones that caused insulin resistance from the placenta.

7. If her glucose challenge test (GCT, a screening test) is 140 mg/dL or higher, she needs the diagnostic 3-hour OGTT to determine whether she has gestational diabetes mellitus. GCT levels of 130 or 135 mg/dL may be used to indicate the need for the diagnostic OGTT test.

8. Releasing tissue after needle insertion; injection over 2 to 4 seconds; quick needle withdrawal

9. These sugars raise blood glucose levels quickly to high levels (hyperglycemia) and alter glucose control for many hours. Correct hypoglycemia with 3 to 4 glucose tablets, ½ cup fruit juice or regular soft drink, 6 crackers, or 1 tablespoon sugar or honey. Refer to p. 665.

10. Rales, dyspnea on exertion, cough, hemoptysis. Progressive edema and tachypnea are added signs.

11. Class III because she has marked symptoms of cardiac decompensation with less than ordinary activity.

12. Anticoagulants of choice include enoxaparin or heparin because these drugs do not cross the placenta.

13. Each labor contraction causes up to 500 mL of blood to be shifted from the uterus and placenta to the central circulation. Approximately 500 mL of blood returns to the central circulation when the placenta delivers. The added blood volume increases the abnormal heart's workload and can result in congestive heart failure.

14. Her excessive weight gain may be caused by any of several factors or a combination of factors: excess food, fluid retention from cardiac decompensation with edema, excess salt intake, or preeclampsia (see Chapter 25). Thus you must assess her diet and assess for other signs and symptoms of cardiac decompensation and preeclampsia, such as hypertension, proteinuria, edema, dyspnea, and hyperactive reflexes.

15. Folic acid is needed for DNA synthesis, a prerequisite for cell duplication and the growth of the fetus and placenta. Folic acid deficiency is associated with a higher incidence of neural tube defects. Getting the required pregnancy amount of folic acid by diet alone is difficult, and folic acid is often destroyed by cooking.

16. Prematurity and intrauterine growth restriction increase fetal morbidity and mortality.

17. Temporary cessation of bone marrow function, jaundice, severe pain in joints and major organs; proneness to pyelonephritis, bone infection, and heart disease

18. Increased spontaneous abortion and fetal death in first trimester. After first trimester, prognosis is good for live birth if there is no active disease. Neonate is vulnerable to permanent congenital heart block that requires a pacemaker.

19. Many anticonvulsants are associated with significant fetal abnormalities and coagulation abnormalities; yet without the drugs, seizures are more likely to occur. Generalized seizures may cause fetal hypoxia, acidosis, and death.

20. (a) Early (acute) stage: flulike symptoms for a few weeks, followed by seroconversion a few weeks or months later. (b) Middle (asymptomatic) period: low-level viral replication and loss of CD4 cells. (c) Transitional period: symptomatic disease. (d) Late (crisis) period: symptomatic disease

21. Use the information in the text, pp. 678-682, to complete this table.
22. AIDS is said to occur when the immune system no longer protects the person and opportunistic infections occur. This occurs during stages 3 and 4 of HIV infection.
23. Zidovudine (recommended for pregnant women) in a multidrug regimen. Other drug classes in therapy may include nucleotide analogs, nucleoside analogs, reverse transcriptase inhibitors, and protease inhibitors.
24. Support grieving and retention of client control; promote wellness (nutrition, rest, activity, avoidance of crowds and poor sanitary conditions, skin care); teach that breastfeeding is contraindicated; reinforce medication information; give support related to anxiety about infant's possible HIV-positive status.
25. Use the information in the text, pp. 683-684, to complete this table.

Check Yourself

1, b; 2, b; 3, a; 4, d; 5, a; 6, c; 7, d; 8, a; 9, b; 10, d; 11, c; 12, d

Case Study

1. During early pregnancy, fetal demand for glucose, coupled with maternal nausea and vomiting, tends to cause maternal hypoglycemia. Debra is near the beginning of the second trimester, so increasing resistance to insulin in her cells and more rapid breakdown of insulin occur to make more glucose available to her fetus.
2. Debra will probably need increasing amounts of insulin as her pregnancy progresses. In addition, the goal is to keep her blood glucose level as near to normal as possible, so she will need to test her blood glucose as many as four to six times each day and may take more frequent insulin doses (regular and intermediate acting). Her diet should have 30 kcal/kg/day distributed among three meals and two or more snacks.
3. Routine assessments at each prenatal visit include vital signs and fetal heart rate; assessment of her blood glucose levels (including daily logs); and urinalysis for protein, glucose, and ketones. Glycosylated hemoglobin testing is performed as needed.
4. Tests needed as pregnancy progresses are designed to evaluate placental function and fetal health and maturity. These may include multiple marker screening, ultrasound, "kick counts," nonstress or contraction stress test, biophysical profile, amniotic fluid index, or amniocentesis to evaluate fetal lung maturity.
5. Possible fetal effects include congenital defects, large or small fetal size, and persistent fetal hypoxia. If her diabetic control of glucose is good, fetal effects may be minimal.
6. Labor may be induced or cesarean delivery performed if the fetus shows signs of decreased placental perfusion with hypoxia. While in labor, Debra will have hourly blood glucose evaluations to determine her need for IV infusion of regular insulin or glucose. Tight glucose control during labor minimizes newborn hypoglycemia.
7. The neonatal nurse should anticipate possible newborn hypoglycemia if the newborn was exposed to high maternal blood glucose in utero, with high fetal insulin secretion to metabolize the glucose. After birth, the glucose supply is cut off while the pancreas continues to secrete large quantities of insulin temporarily. This is most likely to occur if Debra's blood glucose levels were often high.
8. The newborn will need frequent blood glucose monitoring for the first few hours after birth. Care for newborn hypoglycemia, hyperbilirubinemia, or respiratory distress syndrome may be required. See Chapter 30 for more information about caring for the infant of a diabetic mother.

Intrapartum Complications

Learning Activities

1. Match each term with its definition (a-g).

_____ Back labor

_____ K-B test

_____ Premature rupture of the membranes (PROM)

_____ Preterm premature rupture of the membranes (PPROM)

_____ Shoulder dystocia

_____ Tocolytic

_____ Turtle sign

a. Delayed or difficult birth of the shoulders after the head has emerged

b. Retraction of fetal head against the mother's perineum after it emerges

c. Intense back pain associated with fetal occiput posterior position

d. Rupture of the membranes before the onset of labor

e. Rupture of the membranes before the end of week 37

f. Medication to stop preterm or hypertonic uterine contractions

g. Identifying presence of fetal erythrocytes into maternal circulation

2. What are three characteristics of effective uterine activity?

   a.

   b.

   c.

3. Complete the following table to compare the characteristics of hypotonic and hypertonic labor dysfunction.

	Hypotonic Dysfunction	*Hypertonic Dysfunction*
Contraction characteristics		
Uterine resting tone		
Phase of labor when it is most common		
Therapeutic management/nursing care		

4. Why are nursing measures to manage stress and anxiety important in caring for women with either hypotonic or hypertonic labor dysfunction? List some nursing measures. Give examples of nursing measures you use to help a client manage stress and anxiety, whether in the maternity setting or another setting.

5. What is the central principle of nursing actions when dysfunctional labor is a result of ineffective maternal pushing?

6. Why are upright positions good for women who have ineffective second-stage pushing?

7. List nursing measures to promote normal labor when maternal pushing is ineffective for each reason listed.
   a. Fear of injury

   b. Epidural block analgesia

   c. Exhaustion

8. Why are upright maternal positions best to relieve persistent occiput posterior positions? List positions that may be effective, including those other than upright. Have you seen any of these used, including yourself, a family member or friend, or a client cared for in a clinical situation?

9. List four intrapartum problems that are more likely if a woman has a multifetal pregnancy.

a.

b.

c.

d.

10. What are the expected average rates for dilation and fetal descent for the following women after the active phase of labor has been reached?
a. Nulliparas

b. Parous women

11. List nursing measures for a woman having prolonged labor and for her fetus.
a. Maternal

b. Fetal

12. List nursing measures that can be used when a woman has precipitate labor.
a. Promoting fetal oxygenation

b. Promoting maternal comfort

13. What factors may make a woman think her membranes have ruptured when they have not?

14. What care should you plan for a woman whose membranes ruptured at 32 weeks? The fluid was clear, and her vital signs and the fetal heart rate are currently normal. Is there any teaching you should do to help her avoid stimulating preterm labor contractions?

15. List side effects that may occur with beta-adrenergic drugs, such as terbutaline.

16. How do the following drugs stop preterm labor? Give an example of each.
   a. Prostaglandin synthesis inhibitors

   b. Calcium channel blockers

17. What are the primary nursing assessments related to each of these drugs used in the treatment of preterm labor?
   a. Terbutaline

   b. Magnesium sulfate

   c. Indomethacin

   d. Nifedipine

   e. Corticosteroids

18. What are the three variations of prolapsed cord?

a.

b.

c.

19. What are the two objectives if umbilical cord prolapse occurs or is suspected? Why should the nurse avoid handling the prolapsed cord?

20. Describe three variations of uterine rupture.

a.

b.

c.

21. Why is it important that the nurse not push on the uncontracted uterine fundus after birth? What is the correct procedure?

22. Why can anaphylactoid syndrome result in disseminated intravascular coagulation?

23. What are the priorities during the initial treatment of a pregnant woman who had a traumatic injury?

Check Yourself

1. A woman with an otherwise uncomplicated pregnancy is very frustrated because of hypotonic labor. What nursing measure is most appropriate for her?
  a. Do not allow any oral intake.
  b. Start oxytocin at a low rate.
  c. Offer her a warm shower or bath.
  d. Reassure her that her problem is common.

2. A woman has shoulder dystocia when giving birth. The nurse should expect
  a. Immediate forceps delivery
  b. Application of suprapubic pressure
  c. Oxytocin labor augmentation
  d. Turning into a hands-and-knees position

3. While the woman laboring with a twin pregnancy is in bed, a good position for her is
  a. Supine
  b. Hands and knees
  c. Knee-chest
  d. Side-lying

4. Choose the primary nursing measure to promote fetal descent.
  a. Remind the woman to empty her bladder every 1 to 2 hours.
  b. Assist fetal head rotation while doing a vaginal examination.
  c. Have the woman push at least three times with each contraction.
  d. Promote intake of glucose-containing fluids during labor.

5. An infant weighing 3912 g (8 lb, 10 oz) is born vaginally. Shoulder dystocia occurred at birth. Because of this problem, the nurse should assess the infant for
  a. Head swelling that does not extend beyond the skull bone
  b. Inward turning of the feet or legs
  c. Creaking sensation when the clavicles are palpated
  d. Limited abduction of one or both hips

6. A woman is fully dilated, and the fetal station is 0. The fetus is in a right occiput posterior position. She is using Lamaze breathing techniques only. Choose the ideal maternal position for pushing.
  a. Squatting
  b. Left side-lying
  c. Hands and knees
  d. Semisitting

7. A woman is having very rapid labor with her fourth child. What nursing measure is most appropriate to help her manage pain?
  a. Offer butorphanol (Stadol) when she reaches 5 cm cervical dilation.
  b. Keep her in an upright position until full cervical dilation.
  c. Avoid vaginal examinations during the peak of a contraction.
  d. Coach her to use breathing techniques with each contraction as it occurs.

8. Choose the nursing assessment that most clearly suggests intrauterine infection.
   a. Fetal heart rate of 145 to 155 beats per minute (bpm)
   b. Cloudy amniotic fluid
   c. Maternal temperature of 37.8° C (100° F)
   d. Increased bloody show

9. A woman phones the labor unit and says she has been having back discomfort all day. She is at 32 weeks of gestation. The nurse should tell the woman that she
   a. Is having discomfort that is typical of the third trimester
   b. Should come to the hospital if she has increased vaginal drainage
   c. Can increase her fluid intake to reduce Braxton Hicks contractions
   d. Should come to the hospital for further evaluation

10. A woman is receiving magnesium sulfate to stop preterm labor. In addition to fetal heart rate, the essential nursing assessment related to this drug is
    a. For intensity and duration of uterine contractions
    b. Hourly vital signs, heart sounds, and lung sounds
    c. For presence of fetal movements with contractions
    d. Vaginal examination for cervical dilation, effacement, and station

11. A few minutes after a woman's membranes rupture during labor, the fetal heart rate drops from an average of 140 to 150 bpm to 75 to 80 bpm. The priority nursing action is to
    a. Phone the physician to report the fetal heart rate
    b. Assess for other signs that indicate chorioamnionitis
    c. Perform a vaginal examination and palpate for prolapsed cord
    d. Insert an indwelling catheter to assess fluid balance

12. A woman phones the labor unit saying that she has had an abrupt onset of pain between her shoulder blades that is worse when she breathes in. She is scheduled to have a repeat cesarean birth in 1 week. The nurse should
    a. Ask her whether she has had a recent upper respiratory infection
    b. Explain that the growing fetus reduces space to breathe
    c. Have her palpate her uterus for frequent contractions
    d. Tell her that she should come to the hospital promptly

13. Choose the nursing assessment that most clearly suggests hypovolemia.
    a. Urine output of 20 mL/hr
    b. Fetal heart rate of 155 to 165 bpm
    c. Blood pressure of 108/84 mm Hg
    d. Maternal heart rate of 90 to 100 bpm

Developing Insight

1. During clinical practice, observe and discuss with nurses what measures they use for women having back labor.

2. Practice the positions listed for back labor so that you will be familiar with them during clinical practice.

3. If you had to be on bed rest at home for preterm labor, possibly for 6 weeks, what adjustments would you and your family have to make to achieve that recommendation for extended rest? What would be the single most significant obstacle in adhering to bed rest in your life? What type of quiet activities could you do while restricting common activities?

Case Study 1

Ann is admitted at 33 weeks of gestation saying that she thinks her "water broke." This is her fourth pregnancy. Two of her infants were preterm, born at 32 and 27 weeks of gestation, and she has had one termination of pregnancy (elective abortion). She has had regular prenatal care since 6 weeks of gestation.

1. What are the most important additional assessments that the nurse should make?

The nurse notes that a small amount of fluid with a strong odor is draining from Ann's vagina. Using a speculum examination to obtain fluid, the pH test turns blue-black on contact with the fluid, and a fern test is positive. Maternal vital signs are temperature, 37.2° C (99° F); pulse, 86 bpm; respirations, 22 breaths per minute; and blood pressure, 132/80 mm Hg. The fetal heart rate is 162 to 170 bpm. Ann occasionally has a contraction lasting 20 to 30 seconds.

2. What data from the aforementioned assessments are most relevant?

3. What is the main judgment you would make from these data? What is the basis for that judgment?

4. Would you perform a vaginal examination at this point? Why or why not?

Case Study 2

Shawna is an 18-year-old primigravida admitted to the birth center at 27 weeks of gestation in probable preterm labor. Her membranes are intact. The physician writes the following orders:

- Nothing by mouth (NPO) except ice chips or clear fluids
- Complete blood count
- Catheterized urine for routine analysis and culture and sensitivity
- Intravenous (IV) fluids: Ringer's lactate at 200 ml/hr for 1 hour, then 125 ml/hr
- Routine fetal monitoring and maternal vital signs

1. What position is appropriate for Shawna? Why?

2. What is the purpose for a urinalysis and a urine culture and sensitivity?

Shawna will receive magnesium sulfate for tocolysis.

3. What nursing observations are essential in relationship to magnesium sulfate? Why?

Contractions stop, and Shawna will begin taking oral terbutaline.

4. What nursing observations are essential related to use of oral terbutaline?

ANSWERS TO SELECTED QUESTIONS

Learning Activities

1. c, g, d, e, a, f, b
2. Uterine contractions must be (a) coordinated, (b) strong enough, and (c) numerous enough to propel the fetus through the woman's pelvis.
3. Use Table 27-1, p. 695, in the text to complete this question.
4. Hypotonic dysfunction may cause anxiety because the woman expects to be progressing faster; hypertonic dysfunction is stressful because of the near constant discomfort without significant progress. The stress response, associated with anxiety and fear, causes secretion of catecholamines and consumption of glucose, which interfere with normal uterine contraction. Nursing measures include therapeutic communication, pain relief, promotion of relaxation and rest, and positioning.
5. All nursing actions center on helping the woman make each push most effective. Examples include laboring down or delayed pushing, pushing with every other contraction, use of upright positions to push, explaining the expected sensations, coaching her if she cannot feel the urge to push, and reassuring her that there is not an absolute deadline for delivery.
6. They add the force of gravity to maternal pushes.
7. (a) Help the woman understand that her tissues can distend to accommodate the fetus; apply warm compresses to the perineum. (b) Coach her about when to push and stop pushing if she cannot feel contractions well. Help her understand that effective pain management by any method, including nonpharmacologic, promotes progress of labor. (c) Teach the woman to push only when she feels the urge or with every other contraction; administer fluids as ordered; offer reassurance.
8. Upright positions favor fetal descent (gravity) and, with that descent, fetal head rotation. Effective positions for pushing may include squatting, semisitting, side-lying, pushing on toilet, and/or lunging.
9. (In any order) (a) Uterine overdistention with hypotonic dysfunction; (b) abnormal fetal presentation(s); (c) fetal hypoxia; (d) postpartum hemorrhage caused by uterine overdistention
10. (a) Dilation at least 1.2 cm/hr, descent at least 1.0 cm/hr. (b) Dilation at least 1.5 cm/hr, descent at least 2.0 cm/hr.
11. (a) Promotion of comfort, conservation of energy, emotional support, position changes that favor normal progress, and assessments for infection. (b) Observation for signs of intrauterine infection and for compromised fetal oxygenation.

12. (a) Place her in a side-lying position, administer oxygen, maintain blood volume with nonoxytocin IV fluids, stop oxytocin if in use, administer terbutaline or other tocolytic drug that may be ordered. (b) Help woman focus on nonpharmacologic pain-control methods if analgesia is not possible or has not yet taken effect; remain with the woman.
13. Urinary incontinence, increased vaginal discharge, loss of the mucous plug
14. See the text, pp. 705-706, to complete this exercise.
15. Maternal and fetal tachycardia, decreased blood pressure, wide pulse pressure, dysrhythmias, myocardial ischemia, chest pain, pulmonary edema, hyperglycemia and hypokalemia, headache, tremors, and restlessness
16. (a) Block the action of prostaglandins, which stimulate uterine contractions; an example is indomethacin (Indocin). (b) Block the action of calcium, which is necessary for muscle contraction; an example is nifedipine (Adalat, Procardia).
17. (a) Observe maternal blood pressure, pulse, and respirations and fetal heart rate to identify tachycardia or hypotension; assess lung sounds; assess for presence of dyspnea or chest pain to identify pulmonary edema or myocardial ischemia; obtain ordered glucose and potassium levels. (b) Observe for urine output of at least 30 mL/hr, presence of deep tendon reflexes, and respirations of at least 12 breaths per minute; assess heart and lung sounds; observe bowel sounds and assess for constipation; have calcium gluconate available. (c) Observe for nausea, vomiting, heartburn, skin rash, and prolonged bleeding; observe for signs of infection other than fever; check fundal height; have woman do kick counts to identify fetal movements. (d) Teach about flushing of the skin and headache; observe maternal pulse rate (report if over 120 bpm), fetal heart rate, and maternal blood pressure; warn of postural hypotension, and teach woman to assume a sitting or standing position slowly after lying down. (e) Assess lung sounds; teach woman to report chest pain or heaviness or any difficulty in breathing.
18. (a) Occult prolapsed cord cannot be seen or felt on vaginal examination but is suspected based on fetal heart rate. (b) The cord may slip into the vagina, where it can be felt as a pulsating mass during vaginal examination. (c) Complete prolapsed cord slips outside the vagina, where it is visible.
19. Relieve pressure on the cord by any of several measures, including positioning the woman so that her hips are higher than her head and pushing the fetal presenting part upward; increase oxygen delivery to the placenta. Handling the cord may induce arterial spasm in the cord vessels.
20. In any order: (a) Complete rupture—direct communication between the uterine and peritoneal cavities. (b) Incomplete rupture—rupture into the peritoneum or broad

ligament but not into the peritoneal cavity. (c) Dehiscence—partial separation of a previous uterine scar.

21. Pushing on an uncontracted uterus to expel clots after birth may result in uterine inversion. Massage the uterus until it is firm before expelling clots with fundal pressure. Support the lower uterus with one hand just above the symphysis. See also Procedure 17-1, p. 403.

22. Amniotic fluid is rich in thromboplastin, initiating uncontrolled clotting that consumes normal clotting factors.

23. Evaluation and stabilization of maternal injuries; following basic resuscitation rules; arresting hemorrhage; avoiding prolonged supine positioning; evaluating injuries to mother and fetus; expecting large fluid resuscitation needs; providing Rh immune globulin if a fetal-to-maternal hemorrhage is suspected in the Rho(D)-negative woman.

Check Yourself

1, c; 2, b; 3, d; 4, a; 5, c; 6, a; 7, d; 8, b; 9, d; 10, b; 11, c; 12, d; 13, a

Case Study 1

1. The nurse must attempt to verify whether Ann's membranes have ruptured, but without performing a vaginal examination; determine when they ruptured; assess maternal vital signs and fetal heart rate, looking specifically for signs of infection; assess for contractions that may indicate preterm labor as well as preterm premature rupture of membranes.

2. Fluid draining from the vagina; positive pH (7.5) and fern tests; fluid with a strong odor; fetal tachycardia; occasional contraction

3. The vaginal fluid drainage and the positive pH and fern tests suggest that Ann's membranes have ruptured. Infection is suggested by the strong fluid odor and fetal tachycardia. Contractions suggest possible preterm labor.

4. A vaginal examination is not advised at this time because the vaginal discharge is typical of amniotic fluid (meaning that membranes are truly ruptured), there already appears to be an infection, Ann's gestation is preterm, and she is already having contractions. Little information is likely to be gained from the examination, and an examination might introduce more microorganisms into the uterus and may increase contractions. The physician may perform a speculum or vaginal examination or specifically order one.

Case Study 2

1. A side-lying position with the head of the bed low increases placental blood flow and reduces pressure of the fetal presenting part on the cervix. Bed rest may reduce uterine activity.

2. Urinary tract infection is associated with preterm labor and reduces the effectiveness of measures to stop preterm labor.

3. Urine output of at least 30 mL/hr, presence of deep tendon reflexes, and respiratory rate of at least 12 breaths per minute suggest that the magnesium is within safe limits. Serum magnesium levels will also be ordered (see Chapter 25 for additional information).

4. Maintain even spacing of the drug; expect side effects such as palpitations, tremors, restlessness, weakness, or headache. Report heart rate greater than 110 bpm, chest pain, or dyspnea.

CHAPTER 28 Postpartum Maternal Complications

Learning Activities

1. Match each term with its definition (a-h).

_____ Atony

a. A blood clot within a vessel

_____ Embolism

b. A clot or amniotic fluid material forced into smaller vessels by the blood circulation

_____ Petechiae

c. Difference between the systolic and diastolic blood pressure

_____ Placenta accreta

d. Failure of the uterus to return to its prepregnant state in the time expected

_____ Pulse pressure

e. Less-than-normal muscle tone

_____ Subinvolution

f. Placenta that adheres abnormally to the uterine wall

_____ Thrombophlebitis

g. Thrombus formation with inflammation

_____ Thrombus

h. Tiny purplish-red spots on the skin caused by intradermal or submucosal hemorrhage.

2. a. What is the time difference between early and late postpartum hemorrhage?

b. How is hemorrhage defined?

3. What is the most common cause of early postpartum hemorrhage? Describe the pathophysiology of this cause of hemorrhage.

4. How will the nurse recognize uterine atony?

5. What is the correct nursing action if uterine atony is discovered?

6. What signs typically distinguish postpartum hemorrhage caused by uterine atony from hemorrhage caused by lacerations of the birth canal?

7. How do the signs and symptoms of a hematoma differ from those of uterine atony or a bleeding laceration?

8. What discharge teaching related to late postpartum hemorrhage is essential?

9. Why are pregnant and postpartum women prone to develop venous thrombosis?

10. Complete the following chart on venous thrombosis. Include preventive measures.

Condition	Signs and Symptoms	Medical and Nursing Management
Superficial venous thrombosis		
Deep vein thrombosis		

11. What laboratory studies should the nurse expect if the woman is undergoing heparin anticoagulation? If the woman is undergoing warfarin anticoagulation?

12. List client teaching related to long-term anticoagulation.

13. What are the signs and symptoms of pulmonary embolism?

14. What is the definition of *puerperal infection?*

15. What anatomic features of the woman's reproductive tract make infection there potentially serious?

16. What changes of uncomplicated childbirth further increase a woman's risk for reproductive tract infection? What are her protective factors?

17. What signs suggest that a mother may be developing endometritis?

18. List signs and symptoms of wound infection.

19. What liquids can help acidify urine? Why is this acidity helpful in preventing or treating urinary tract infection?

20. Why is it important that the breastfeeding mother with mastitis avoid engorgement?

21. What is the key difference between postpartum blues and postpartum depression?

22. What nursing interventions are appropriate for the woman with postpartum depression?

Check Yourself

1. The nurse notes that a woman has excess lochia 2 hours after vaginal birth of an 8-lb baby. The priority nursing action is to
 a. Catheterize her to check urine output
 b. Check her blood pressure, pulse, and respirations
 c. Assess the firmness of her uterus
 d. Notify her physician or nurse-midwife

2. Choose the signs and symptoms that suggest postpartum hemorrhage causing a hematoma.
 a. Rectal pain accompanied by a rising pulse
 b. Cramping accompanied by a steady trickle of blood
 c. Soft uterine fundus and a falling blood pressure
 d. Heavy lochia accompanied by tachypnea and dyspnea

3. One hour after a woman gives birth vaginally, the nurse notes that her fundus is firm, 2 fingerbreadths above the umbilicus, and deviated to the right. Lochia rubra is moderate. Her perineum is slightly edematous, with no bruising; an ice pack is in place. The priority nursing action is to
 a. Chart these expected normal assessments
 b. Have the woman empty her bladder
 c. Change the perineal ice pack to a warm pack
 d. Increase the rate of the oxytocin infusion

4. What drug should be readily available when a woman is receiving heparin therapy?
 a. Vitamin K
 b. Methylergonovine
 c. Ferrous sulfate
 d. Protamine sulfate

5. The nurse's initial response if a pulmonary embolism is suspected should be to
   a. Start a second intravenous (IV) line and prepare for transfusion
   b. Raise the head of the bed and administer oxygen
   c. Insert a catheter to monitor urine output
   d. Lower the head of the bed and elevate the legs

6. A woman has an 8-lb, 9-oz baby after an 18-hour labor that required a vacuum extraction. Her membranes have been ruptured for 15 hours. Based on these facts, client teaching should emphasize
   a. Reporting foul-smelling lochia and fever
   b. Delaying intercourse for at least 6 weeks
   c. Eating a diet that is high in iron and vitamin C
   d. Losing weight over at least a 6-month period

7. Postpartum teaching related to urinary health should emphasize
   a. Drinking any type of fluid whenever thirsty
   b. Allowing the bladder to fill to promote emptying
   c. Cleansing the perineum in a front-to-back direction
   d. Eating two servings of acidic fruits or vegetables each day

8. A new father tells a nurse friend that his wife is agitated and acting bizarrely. She says she hears voices. Her baby is 2 weeks old. The father is concerned about the care the mother is giving the baby. The nurse should
   a. Tell the father that this is just severe postpartum blues and will pass in a few days if he shows enough support
   b. Suggest the father try talking to his wife to find out what is bothering her about being a new mother
   c. Explain that the mother will probably need psychotherapy and refer him to support groups for postpartum depression
   d. Tell the father to call the physician immediately and not to leave the woman alone with the baby

9. A breastfeeding woman develops mastitis. She tells the nurse that she will feed her baby formula instead of breastfeeding until the infection is healed. The best nursing response is that
   a. Emptying the breast is important to prevent an abscess
   b. A tight breast binder or bra will help reduce engorgement
   c. She should continue to drink extra fluids while weaning
   d. Breastfeeding can continue when her temperature is normal

10. A woman tells you she has been teary for most of the 2 weeks since the birth of her baby. Although the infant appears to be cared for appropriately, the mother states that she feels too tired to spend as much time with him as she should. She has lost her appetite and cannot sleep at night. She has been too ashamed to tell anyone before now. The nurse's best response is to
   a. Tell her this is normal postpartum blues and she will get over it in a few more days
   b. Suggest she get help to care for the baby and that with more rest she will feel fine
   c. Listen to her feelings carefully and then acknowledge that something is wrong
   d. Suggest she spend time away from the baby to rest from the constant infant care

Developing Insight

1. During clinical practice, review the charts of postpartum women. List all factors that put them at higher risk for infection and the type of infection that would probably occur based on these factors. How should your nursing care change according to their risk for infection or the site of the infection?

2. Use the information in Chapter 9 to plan a diet for a breastfeeding woman who had a postpartum hemorrhage without blood replacement.

3. Get information from one of the resources for postpartum depression listed in your text. Find out what resources are available in your community.

Case Study

Jen is a gravida 1, para 1, who had a vaginal birth of a 9-lb baby 1½ hours ago. Her fundus has remained firm, midline, and 1 fingerbreadth below the umbilicus. She has not yet voided. Vital signs are stable, and she is afebrile. She received 2 tablets of hydrocodone with acetaminophen (Vicodin) for perineal pain 30 minutes after birth. She now requests "something stronger" for pain because the previous analgesic has been ineffective.

1. What are some possible explanations for the ineffectiveness of the analgesic?

2. Does the nurse need more information? If so, what?

The nurse checks Jen's vital signs 30 minutes later. Her blood pressure is near its previous levels, but her pulse is slightly faster. Her fundal height, firmness, and lochia amount are unchanged. Her perineum is intact and has a small amount of edema. She rates her pain as a 7 on a 1 to 10 pain scale. The nurse replaces the ice pack to the perineum that has been in place since Jen's recovery period began.

3. Are any other interventions warranted? If so, what are they and why are they appropriate?

ANSWERS TO SELECTED QUESTIONS

Learning Activities

1. e, b, h, f, c, d, g, a
2. (a) Early postpartum hemorrhage occurs within 24 hours of birth; late hemorrhage occurs after 24 hours or up to 6 to 12 weeks after birth. (b) Hemorrhage may be defined as loss of more than 500 mL of blood after vaginal birth, loss of more than 1000 mL of blood after cesarean birth, a decrease in hematocrit of 10% or more, or a need for blood transfusion.
3. Uterine atony is the most common cause. It occurs when the muscle fibers of the uterus do not contract firmly to compress bleeding endometrial vessels at the placental site.
4. The uterus is difficult to locate, and when found it is soft rather than firm and higher than the expected level near the umbilicus. It may become firm with massage but may fail to remain firm. Lochia and clots are excessive.
5. Support the lower uterus with one hand while using the other hand to gently but firmly massage the fundus until it contracts. Press down on the fundus toward the vagina *after the uterus is firm* to express clots that have accumulated in the uterine cavity and could interfere with continued uterine contraction. Check for a distended bladder, often indicated when the uterus is displaced to one side (usually the right). Have the woman urinate or catheterize her if necessary. Maintain intravenous access. If the problem continues, notify the health care provider. The physician may order drugs such as oxytocin, methylergonovine, prostaglandin F_{2alpha}, Prostin E2, or misoprostol to maintain uterine contraction.
6. Excess, usually brighter red, bleeding that may be heavy or slow but steady in the presence of a firmly contracted uterus that is in the expected location suggests a laceration.
7. With hematoma, pain is the greatest distinction, because confined bleeding exerts pressure on sensory nerves. The uterus is firm, excluding uterine atony as the cause. Lochia is normal because the bleeding is concealed, excluding a bleeding laceration. A bulging, discolored mass may be visible. A rising pulse and respiratory rate and falling blood pressure are signs of hypovolemia that may occur with any type of hemorrhage.
8. Women should be told the normal sequence, amount, and duration of lochia. They should be taught assessment and expected descent of the fundus. Guidelines should be provided for reporting deviations from normal.
9. They have stasis of blood in the veins of the lower extremities and have higher levels of clotting factors and suppression of factors that prevent clot formation. Injury to the vessels may occur during birth.
10. Refer to text, pp. 740-743, to complete this chart.
11. Standard unfractionated heparin: activated partial thromboplastin time (aPTT) and platelets. Warfarin: international normalized ratio (INR).
12. Teach heparin injection technique to client and a family member, as appropriate. Teach client to report unusual bruising or petechiae, nosebleeds, blood in urine or stools, bleeding gums, or increased vaginal bleeding. Instruct her to use a soft toothbrush and not to go barefoot. Explain side effects of the specific anticoagulant. Caution about drug interactions and avoiding alcohol. Teach when to return for laboratory studies. Teach client to avoid large amounts of foods high in vitamin K if taking warfarin.
13. Signs and symptoms vary according to the degree of pulmonary blood flow obstruction, but include dyspnea, chest pain, tachycardia, tachypnea, rales, cough, hemoptysis, abdominal pain, low grade fever, and decreased oxygen saturation and partial pressure of oxygen. Atelectasis and pleural effusion may be seen on x-ray films.
14. Puerperal infection is an infection that is associated with childbirth, in which the woman has a fever of 38°C (100.4° F) or higher after the first 24 hours, occurring on at least 2 days during the first 10 days following birth.
15. All the parts of the female reproductive tract are connected to each other and to the peritoneal cavity. The area is richly supplied with blood vessels and lymphatics, providing a well-nourished, dark, warm environment that favors bacterial growth.
16. Amniotic fluid, blood, and lochia make the normally acidic vagina more alkaline, fostering growth of organisms. The necrotic endometrial lining and lochia promote growth of anaerobic organisms. Small areas of trauma allow microorganisms to enter the tissues. However, granulocytes in the endometrium and lochia help prevent infection.
17. Fever, lochia with a foul odor, chills, anorexia, cramping, uterine tenderness, malaise, tachycardia, subinvolution
18. Edema, warmth, redness, pain, separation of edges, seropurulent drainage
19. Apricot, plum, prune, and cranberry juices help acidify urine, which makes the urine less friendly to microorganisms.
20. Engorgement causes stasis of milk, which promotes growth of infecting microorganisms, possibly leading to abscess.
21. Postpartum depression symptoms are more intense and persistent (lasting at least 2 weeks) than those of

postpartum blues, which is temporary and mild. Symptoms of postpartum depression include changes in appetite, weight, sleep, and psychomotor activity; decreased energy; feelings of worthlessness or guilt; difficulty thinking, concentrating, or making decisions; or recurrent thoughts of death or suicide, plans or attempts.

22. Help the woman express her feelings and identify stressors; discuss methods to relieve stress, such as relaxation techniques; model ways to respond to the infant; teach the family what to expect and how to help the mother; refer to physician for psychotherapy and medications; and refer to support groups.

Check Yourself

1, c; 2, a; 3, b; 4, d; 5, b; 6, a; 7, c; 8, d; 9, a; 10, c

Case Study

1. The medication could be taking longer than usual to exert its analgesic properties, it could be outdated, Jen's pain tolerance at this time could be very low, or other birth trauma may have occurred. In addition, although Jen's fundal height is appropriate, she may need to urinate because it has been 1½ hours since birth and her bladder may be fuller than it seems.

2. The nurse needs more information about the pain: location, intensity on a 1 to 10 scale (comparing its present level with the level before she took the analgesic), character, and if anything worsens or improves it. In addition, the nurse must look at Jen's perineal area for evidence of a hematoma.

3. If Jen still has not voided, the nurse should carefully assess her bladder and place her on the bedpan to void. However, Jen's symptoms suggest a concealed hemorrhage with early hypovolemia: unrelieved pain and a rising pulse in the presence of a firm fundus and normal lochia. Unrelieved pain is not typical of a full bladder, although it may worsen the pain of a hematoma. Therefore, Jen should not ambulate to the bathroom because of the higher risk of fainting. If she does not void promptly, it would be appropriate to catheterize her (assuming there is an order), both to determine whether emptying her bladder relieves the pain and to determine her urine output, which is an indicator of fluid volume status. The physician or nurse-midwife should be notified promptly of all assessments and interventions.

High-Risk Newborn: Complications Associated with Gestational Age and Development

---

Learning Activities

1. Match each term with its definition (a-e).

_____ Corrected age

_____ Kangaroo care

_____ Residual

_____ Silverman-Andersen index

_____ Surfactant

a. Substance in the alveoli that reduces surface tension

b. Tool to evaluate the degree of respiratory distress

c. Holding an infant skin-to-skin

d. Chronologic age minus weeks born prematurely

e. Formula in the stomach before a gavage feeding

2. Classify each of these newborn physical characteristics as (pt) preterm, (t) term, or (pm) postmature. Some characteristics will have more than one answer.

a. _____ Underdeveloped flexor muscles

b. _____ Abundant hair on the head

c. _____ Loose skin

d. _____ Little or no lanugo

e. _____ Poor muscle tone

f. _____ Long fingernails

g. _____ Visible blood vessels on the abdomen

h. _____ Long, thin body

i. _____ Creases covering the entire sole

j. _____ Alert and wide-eyed

k. _____ Little subcutaneous fat

l. _____ Dry and peeling skin

m. _____ "Frog leg" position

n. _____ Meconium staining

o. _____ Abundant vernix caseosa

p. _____ Full areola 5 to 10 mm

q. _____ Soft, flexible ears

r. _____ Labia majora covering clitoris and labia minora

3. Explain newborn classifications of gestational age and birth-weight.
   a. Late preterm

   b. Preterm

   c. Low birth-weight

   d. Very low birth-weight

   e. Extremely low birth-weight

   f. Intrauterine growth–restricted

4. List at least five problems common to late preterm infants.

5. Distinguish periodic breathing from apneic spells.
   a. Periodic breathing

   b. Apneic spells

6. Why is the prone position not advised for normal newborns, but good for the preterm infant?

7. Describe five major disadvantages the preterm infant has in regulating temperature.

8. List common measures to help the preterm infant maintain thermoregulation.

9. What factors make fluid and electrolyte balance difficult in the preterm infant?

10. Describe measures to evaluate fluid status in the preterm infant.

11. List signs of dehydration and overhydration.
   a. Dehydration

   b. Overhydration

12. How can the nurse reduce trauma to the preterm infant's skin?

13. What factors typically increase a preterm infant's risk for infection?

14. How can the nurse help an infant during painful procedures?

15. What are the possible reasons that a preterm infant may need gavage feedings instead of nipple feedings?

16. List four methods to identify intestinal complications.

17. What is the purpose of giving an infant a pacifier when gavage feeding?

18. What advantages do breastfeeding and breast milk have for the preterm infant?

19. What signs suggest development of respiratory distress syndrome?

20. What signs of necrotizing enterocolitis should the nurse report to the physician?

21. What are the two possible consequences for a fetus who is postmature?
    a.

    b.

22. Why is the postmature infant likely to have problems with hypoglycemia and thermoregulation?

a. Hypoglycemia

b. Thermoregulation

Check Yourself

1. When feeding an infant who was born at 35 6/7 weeks of gestation, the nurse will expect the infant to be likely to
a. Require intravenous feedings
b. Have a weak suck and fall asleep
c. Suck vigorously but regurgitate more often
d. Be unable to feed at the mother's breast

2. After a stressful procedure on a 4-lb, 2-oz infant, the nurse should
a. Feed the baby breast milk or formula
b. Place the baby in a supine position
c. Allow the baby to rest undisturbed
d. Delay the next feeding for an hour

3. The purpose of containment in care of the preterm infant is to
a. Simulate the enclosed uterine environment when stressful procedures must be performed
b. Gradually reduce the percentage of supplemental oxygen needed to prevent hypoxia
c. Prevent insensible water loss from the large skin surface area of preterm infants
d. Limit the formula given by gavage feedings as the infant starts nipple feeding

4. Discharge teaching for the parents of an infant with bronchopulmonary dysplasia should emphasize
a. That recurrent grunting and retractions are common
b. The importance of providing enzyme formula supplements
c. Careful handling to prevent pulmonary hemorrhage
d. Managing equipment for oxygen supplementation

5. Nursing care that reduces the risk for periventricular or intraventricular hemorrhage includes
a. Assessing for abnormal heart rhythms or murmurs
b. Handling the infant minimally and gently
c. Providing stimulation to enhance brain function
d. Supplementing with high levels of oxygen

6. For the infant who is postmature, what should be expected during the first 8 to 12 hours after birth?
a. Blood glucose determinations
b. Placement under phototherapy
c. Surfactant replacement
d. Blood transfusions

7. A preterm infant has been receiving breast milk by gavage every 3 hours. The nurse checks the residual before giving the next feeding and finds it equals most of the last feeding. The nurse should
a. Decrease the amount of milk by 2 mL/kg
b. Add extra fortifier to the breast milk feeding
c. Delay the feeding for 1 hour and recheck the residual
d. Hold the feeding and notify the physician

8. The mother of a preterm infant weighing 1200 g is worried because her baby does not seem to respond to her. The nurse's best response is that
   a. She should stroke her baby, as well as talk to him
   b. Infants this young cannot sense the presence of others
   c. Her baby is too immature to tolerate much stimulation
   d. The baby will respond to her better just before feeding

9. When a medically fragile infant is going to be discharged, the nurse should
   a. Assist the parents to notify the utility companies
   b. Suggest parents employ a full-time RN or CNA
   c. Advise parents to have two of each kind of equipment they will use
   d. Help parents arrange for care in an extended care facility

10. The nurse is preparing to feed a growing preterm infant. The infant is restless and fussy. She sucks on her fingers and a pacifier well. She has had no problems with regurgitation of breast milk. Vital signs are temperature, 98.7° F; pulse, 156 beats per minute (bpm); respirations, 70 breaths per minute. Oxygen saturation is 96%. The nurse should
    a. Suggest that the mother try to breastfeed
    b. Wait until the infant is more awake to feed
    c. Feed the infant breast milk by gavage tube
    d. Help the mother feed the infant by bottle

Developing Insight

1. During clinical practice, assess the gestational age of infants you care for and plot their weight, length, and head circumference on a chart to classify them as small for gestational age (SGA), appropriate for gestational age (AGA), or large for gestational age (LGA). Identify those who have intrauterine growth restriction (IUGR) and determine what type of IUGR exists (symmetric or asymmetric).

2. Note sources of environmental stress for sick or normal newborns in the hospital. How might these stresses be reduced without compromising other care?

3. Talk with parents whose preterm infant is now at home. Ask what was helpful to them while their baby was in the hospital.

Case Study

Kaylee was born 3 weeks ago at 32 weeks of gestation. Her mother had placenta previa. Continued bleeding along with persistent contractions required a cesarean birth. Kaylee weighed 1642 g (3 lb, 10 oz) at birth. She has made good progress and requires minimal supplemental oxygen. Although she lost weight at first, she has regained her birth-weight and is gaining approximately 25 g each day. She is fed breast milk by a combination of gavage with bottle feeding or breastfeeding. She sometimes has difficulty maintaining her body temperature, but this is improving.

1. What are the three priority nursing diagnoses that are likely in this scenario? What factors support the nursing diagnoses?
   a.

   b.

   c.

2. What nursing interventions can help Kaylee's parents feel that she is indeed *their* baby?

ANSWERS TO SELECTED QUESTIONS

Learning Activities

1. d, c, e, b, a
2. a, pt; b, t or pm; c, pm; d, pm; e, pt; f, pm; g, pt; h, pm; i, t or pm; j, pm; k, pt or pm; l, t or pm; m, pt; n, pm; o, pt; p, t or pm; q, pt; r, t or pm
3. (a) Born between 34 0/7 and 36 6/7 weeks of gestation; (b) born before the 38th week of gestation begins; (c) birth-weight 2500 g (5 lb, 8 oz) or less; (d) birth-weight 1500 g (3 lb, 5 oz) or less; (e) birth-weight 1000 g (2 lb, 3 oz) or less; (f) birth-weight and growth less than expected for duration of gestation
4. Respiratory distress syndrome, transient tachypnea of the newborn, apnea of prematurity, inadequate thermoregulation, hypoglycemia, hyperbilirubinemia, kernicterus, seizures, feeding difficulties, neurodevelopmental disorders, rehospitalization after discharge
5. (a) Periodic breathing is lack of breathing for 5 to 10 seconds without cyanosis or bradycardia, which may be followed by rapid respirations for 10 to 15 seconds. (b) Apneic spells usually last 20 seconds or longer along with cyanosis or bradycardia.
6. The prone position is associated with an increased incidence of sudden infant death syndrome (SIDS). However, for the preterm infant the prone position reduces energy used for respirations, increases oxygenation, enhances respiratory control, and improves mechanics and volume. Preterm infants should be moved to the prone position as soon as they can tolerate it.
7. (a) Thin skin with little insulating fat; (b) accumulation of less heat-producing brown fat; (c) poor flexion to reduce exposed body surfaces; (d) proportionally more body surface area than full-term infant; (e) immature temperature control center in the brain
8. Radiant warmers, incubators, warmed oxygen, measures to reduce air currents, transparent plastic blanket over the radiant warmer bed, keeping portholes of incubators closed as much as possible, hats and heated blankets when out of the incubator or radiant warmer, kangaroo care, padding surfaces with warmed blankets when procedures are performed
9. Greater water loss through the thin, permeable skin; nonflexed positioning and large surface area that increases insensible losses; drying effects of outside heat sources; rapid respiratory rate and use of oxygen; poor ability of kidneys to concentrate or dilute urine; poor ability of kidneys to regulate electrolytes
10. Calculating intake and output: weighing diapers to determine the difference between the dry weight and the wet weight; collecting urine with cotton balls at the perineum to check specific gravity; weighing the unclothed infant daily or twice daily on the same scale at the same time of day; observation of signs of dehydration or overhydration
11. (a) Dehydration: urine output <1 mL/kg/hr; increased urine specific gravity; excessive weight loss; dry skin or mucous membranes; sunken fontanel; poor tissue turgor; increased blood sodium, protein, and hematocrit; hypotension. (b) Overhydration: urine output >3 mL/kg/hr with decreased specific gravity; edema; too-rapid weight gain; bulging fontanel; decreased blood sodium, protein, and hematocrit; moist lung sounds; dyspnea.
12. Avoid adhesive tape. Instead, use gauze wraps or products that are easy to remove from the skin, pectin or hydrocolloid barriers, transparent semipermeable dressings, hydrogel or silicone-based adhesives, or hydrocolloid sheet dressings; avoid cleansing products that are traumatic and rinse with sterile water or saline; apply emollients to lessen water loss from the skin; position the infant to avoid pressure and change positions frequently; use humidity in incubators to decrease drying the skin
13. Maternal infection, incomplete passive antibody transfer from the mother, immature immune response, invasive therapeutic procedures that damage delicate skin, exposure to organisms in the hospital
14. Use a pain scale to assess pain level (changes in pulse, respirations, blood pressure, oxygen saturation, or color; crying or "cry face"), use containment and facilitated tucking; provide rest periods before, during, and after procedures; use pacifiers, sucrose, soft talking, and ordered medication.
15. Poor suck, swallow, and breathing coordination; rapid respirations; immature gag reflex; high expenditure of energy for sucking
16. Check residual before beginning feedings, measure abdominal circumference to identify distention, test stools for reducing substance and occult blood, observe for vomiting or diarrhea.
17. Association of the comfort of fullness with sucking and oral stimulation; preparation for nipple feeding; decreases behavior changes during feedings; brings infant to an alert state
18. Breast milk has immunologic benefits; it is more easily digested; it provides enzymes, hormones, and growth factors; it helps prevent infections and necrotizing enterocolitis; it causes less stress because the baby can better regulate respirations and suckling; the mother's body keeps the baby warm.
19. Grunting on expiration, tachypnea, tachycardia, nasal flaring, retractions, cyanosis, rales or decreased breath sounds, acidosis with hypoxemia; chest x-ray films show "ground glass" appearance or atelectasis
20. Any of these signs should be reported: increased abdominal girth due to distention (rather than growth),

increased or bile-stained gastric residuals, decreased or absent bowel sounds, bowel loops seen through the abdominal wall, vomiting, abdominal tenderness, signs of infection, blood in the stools.

21. (a) Placental deterioration with chronic hypoxia, malnutrition, oligohydramnios, cord compression, meconium passage into the amniotic fluid, asphyxia at birth, higher perinatal mortality. (b) Continued placental function, with continued growth that increases the risk for birth injury or cesarean birth.

22. (a) Poor glycogen stores at birth; (b) little insulating subcutaneous fat

Check Yourself

1, b; 2, c; 3, a; 4, d; 5, b; 6, a; 7, d; 8, c; 9, a; 10, c

Case Study

1. The most likely nursing diagnoses are as follows: (a) "Risk for Ineffective Infant Feeding Pattern related to fatigue when nippling"; (b) "Risk for Ineffective Thermoregulation related to immaturity of temperature regulation and minimal body fat"; and (c) "Risk for Impaired Attachment" related to prolonged separation of parents from hospitalized infant.

2. Point out how Kaylee has begun to gain weight. Emphasize the benefits of the mother's breast milk for a preterm infant, even if some must be given by gavage. Encourage the parents to hold and stroke Kaylee to the limits of her tolerance, and point out when she responds positively to them. Show them signs of overstimulation and explain what this means and how to respond. Involve the parents in her care. Gradually have the parents take over more of her care as you observe unobtrusively. Place her name on the incubator to personalize it. Note her individual responses to care, such as likes and dislikes or amusing habits. Provide visual stimulation (as tolerated) as you would for other newborns. Give parents the phone number to the nursery, and encourage them to call at any time. If available, refer them to a parental support group.

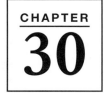

High-Risk Newborn:
Acquired and Congenital
Conditions

Learning Activities

1. Match each term with its definition (a-h).

_____ Exchange transfusion

a. Air leakage into the middle area of the chest between the sternum and vertebral column

_____ Extracorporeal membrane oxygenation

b. Protrusion of meninges and spinal cord through a vertebral defect

_____ Gastroschisis

c. Intestines protruding into the cord

_____ Meningocele

d. Technique to oxygenate the blood while bypassing the lungs

_____ Myelomeningocele

e. Air leakage into the chest cavity

_____ Omphalocele

f. Removal of small amounts of blood and replacement with donor blood

_____ Pneumomediastinum

g. Abdominal defect with intestines protruding out

_____ Pneumothorax

h. Protrusion of meninges through a spinal defect

2. What is the difference between primary and secondary apnea? Which is more ominous? Why?

3. Compare the following newborn respiratory complications.

Parameter	Transient Tachypnea of the Newborn	Meconium Aspiration Syndrome	Persistent Pulmonary Hypertension
Causes			
Manifestations			
Therapeutic management			
Nursing considerations			

4. What is the relationship among bilirubin, jaundice, bilirubin encephalopathy, and kernicterus?

5. Why is phototherapy begun at lower bilirubin levels if the infant is preterm rather than full-term?

6. Formulate a simple explanation about phototherapy to give to parents of a jaundiced newborn. Include in your explanation why the treatment is needed, how it works, and what precautions are needed to prevent injury.

7. What is the purpose of an exchange transfusion?

8. Match the neonatal infections with the statement that fits.

_____ Candidiasis	a. Infants exposed at birth receive immune globulin and immunization to prevent infection.
_____ Chlamydia	b. Typically manifested by white patches in mouth that resemble milk curds.
_____ Cytomegalovirus	c. Intellectual disability is associated with these infections.
_____ Gonorrhea	d. Antibiotics may be given to high-risk mothers in labor or to infant after birth.
_____ Group B streptococcal infection	e. Antibiotic prophylaxis soon after birth can prevent blindness.
_____ Hepatitis B	f. Maternal antiviral treatment during pregnancy can markedly reduce transmission to infant.
_____ Human immunodeficiency virus/acquired immunodeficiency syndrome	g. May cause eye infection or pneumonia.

9. List factors that make newborns more vulnerable to sepsis neonatorum.

10. Compare early- and late-onset neonatal sepsis.

11. How does the newborn manifest infection compared with an older child? Why is it particularly important to identify newborn sepsis early?

12. What tests are usually performed when neonatal sepsis is suspected? What are their purposes and, as appropriate, how do they change in sepsis?

13. Why are tests for drug levels often needed for antibiotics?

14. How can diabetes cause both intrauterine growth restriction and large-for-gestational-age infants?

15. Explain why the following complications occur in infants of diabetic mothers.
  a. Respiratory distress syndrome

  b. Hypoglycemia

  c. Hypocalcemia

  d. Polycythemia

16. Describe the typical appearance of a macrosomic infant of a diabetic mother (IDM).

17. List signs of neonatal hypoglycemia.

18. Why is the infant with polycythemia more likely to need phototherapy?

19. List infant behaviors that should cause a nurse to suspect prenatal drug exposure.

20. What care is appropriate for the infant with neonatal abstinence syndrome?

21. Why are gavage feedings sometimes needed for the drug-exposed infant, even if born at term?

22. What assistance with feeding does the mother of a drug-exposed infant need?

23. Complete the following chart classifying congenital heart defects by blood flow abnormalities.

Abnormality	Description	Example
Increased pulmonary blood flow		
Obstructed blood flow		
Decreased pulmonary blood flow		
Left-to-right shunting defects		

24. Why would giving oxygen not improve cyanosis if the infant has a right-to-left shunt?

Check Yourself

1. An infant is born cyanotic, with poor muscle tone, and gasping respirations. He has been positioned under a radiant warmer, suctioned, dried, and stimulated by rubbing his back. There is little improvement. What should be done next?
   a. Determine the Apgar.
   b. Try flicking the feet to stimulate the infant.
   c. Begin resuscitation.
   d. Reposition the infant.

2. Naloxone for neonatal use is supplied in 1-mg/mL vials. The correct volume of naloxone for a neonate weighing 5 lb, 4 oz is approximately
   a. 0.24 mL
   b. 0.43 mL
   c. 0.5 mL
   d. 0.6 mL

3. If thick meconium is present in the amniotic fluid, the depressed infant has an endotracheal tube inserted and meconium is suctioned. The primary reason for this action is to
   a. Limit transfer of infectious substances to the lungs
   b. Reduce the likelihood of secondary apnea
   c. Prevent persistence of abnormal cardiac shunts
   d. Prevent severe respiratory difficulty after birth

4. Infants receiving phototherapy should be fed every 2 to 3 hours to
   a. Promote excretion of bilirubin from the bowel
   b. Prevent development of low body temperature
   c. Prevent bilirubin-associated weight loss
   d. Decrease abnormal intestinal flora

5. The nurse notes that a 24-hour-old infant is lethargic and his temperature is below normal, a change from an earlier assessment that was normal. His mother states that he did not breastfeed well and that he spit up the small amount he had ingested. The nurse's next action should be to
   a. Reassure the mother that infants are often sluggish this soon after birth.
   b. Assess for signs of sepsis and report assessments to the physician.
   c. Determine whether there is jaundice over the thoracic and abdominal areas.
   d. Feed the infant formula to determine the intake more accurately.

6. A mother who has diabetes is concerned because her 36-hour-old baby is "so yellow." She tells the nurse that she thought her baby's problems were over when his blood glucose stabilized, even though he was smaller than expected. The nurse's response is based on the knowledge that
   a. The baby's liver is much less mature than expected and cannot handle normal red blood cell breakdown.
   b. The baby lived in a low oxygen environment during pregnancy and must eliminate excess red blood cells.
   c. The baby's high blood glucose levels immediately after birth caused a slight dehydration that increases jaundice.
   d. Early feedings slowed elimination of meconium that would have also eliminated excess bilirubin.

7. The nurse notes that a 12-hour-old infant is jittery, but his blood glucose level is normal. The infant seems hungry but takes only 0.25 oz of formula with difficulty. The nurse's next action should be to
   a. Apply a bag to collect the next sample of urine.
   b. Recheck the glucose level 30 minutes after the feeding.
   c. Ask the mother to continue trying to feed the baby.
   d. Swaddle the infant tightly and try to feed more formula.

8. Choose the caregiver teaching that is most appropriate for the infant who was exposed to drugs prenatally.
   a. Breastfeeding is especially important to the infant's recovery.
   b. Hold the baby in an en face position to allow prolonged eye contact.
   c. Swaddle the baby with arms and legs flexed to reduce startling.
   d. Do not burp the baby until at least 1 oz of formula has been taken.

9. An infant has a unilateral cleft lip. The mother expresses her disappointment to the nurse, stating, "I wanted to breastfeed my son because of all the good things that breast milk contains." How should the nurse respond?
   a. "Breastfeeding is often possible because the soft breast fills in the cleft of the lip."
   b. "It may be possible to breastfeed your baby after his lip is surgically repaired."
   c. "It's difficult for you to accept formula feeding after you planned to nurse him."
   d. "Would you like to pump your milk and then give it to the baby in a bottle?"

10. Choose the appropriate nursing care for the infant with myelomeningocele.
    a. Position supine with the head elevated 30 to 45 degrees.
    b. Restrict parent contact to reduce the risk for infection.
    c. Assess for presence of lower-extremity reflexes each shift.
    d. Measure the head circumference during each shift.

Developing Insight

1. Imagine that you are the nurse caring for a baby who needs resuscitation at birth. List the things you would want to have readily available. Write out your actions and what you think the actions of other team members will be from the time the baby is brought to the warmer until he or she is breathing adequately.

2. How might the actions in the previous scenario change if there were thick meconium in the amniotic fluid?

3. Compare an infant of a diabetic mother with other newborns. What similarities and differences do you note? Can any of these be explained by how well the woman's diabetes was controlled during pregnancy?

4. Observe the reception the mother of an infant exposed to drugs prenatally receives when she visits the nursery. Are the nurses' reactions positive or negative? If they are not positive, what nursing actions might better benefit the mother and infant?

Case Study

Steven is 20 hours old. He was born vaginally with forceps after a 16-hour labor. He has bilateral cephalohematomas. His mother has type O, Rh-positive blood, and Steven's blood type is A, Rh-positive. His bilirubin level was 7.5 mg/dL, and his Coombs' test was positive on a cord blood sample. He is slightly jaundiced.

1. Does any of the previous information indicate a pathologic condition?

2. What other assessments should be performed?

At 24 hours after birth, Steven's bilirubin level is 12.5 mg/dL, and his skin is more jaundiced.

3. What treatment does Steven require at this time? How does the treatment affect his bilirubin level?

4. Identify the required nursing interventions for Steven once treatment for jaundice has begun.

5. What are the possible side effects of this phototherapy?

ANSWERS TO SELECTED QUESTIONS

Learning Activities

1. f, d, g, h, b, c, a, e
2. In primary apnea, the infant may respond to stimulation and oxygen when respirations cease. In secondary apnea, the infant does not respond to stimulation and loses consciousness. Secondary apnea is more ominous because stimulation is not enough to reverse it, blood oxygen levels decrease further, and resuscitation must be started immediately to prevent permanent brain damage or death.
3. Refer to text, pp. 801 and 804-806 to complete this question.
4. Bilirubin is the waste product of excess erythrocyte breakdown. Jaundice is the staining of the skin and sclerae by bilirubin. Bilirubin encephalopathy is an acute condition from bilirubin in the brain and may lead to kernicterus. Kernicterus is the chronic and permanent result of toxicity from bilirubin.
5. Bilirubin encephalopathy may occur at lower bilirubin levels in the preterm infant than in the term infant.
6. Refer to text, pp. 807-808, and Nursing Care Plan 30-1 to formulate your explanation.
7. Exchange transfusion replaces the infant's blood that has high levels of bilirubin, unconjugated bilirubin, and sensitized erythrocytes with blood that has normal levels of these components. The blood that replaces the infant's blood is not sensitive to the circulating antibodies from the mother that have destroyed the infant's own erythrocytes.
8. b, g, c, e, d, a, f
9. Immune system immaturity, with a slower reaction to invading organisms; poor localization of infection that allows more extensive spread of infection; less effective blood-brain barrier
10. Early-onset sepsis is related to prolonged rupture of membranes, prolonged labor, or chorioamnionitis; infants have signs within 24 hours of life and the infection progresses more rapidly. Mortality rate is 5% to 20%. Pneumonia and meningitis are common manifestations. Late-onset sepsis develops after the first week. It is more localized and may involve the central nervous system, often with long-term effects. Mortality rate is 5%.
11. Signs of infection are often more subtle in infants than in older children. Signs include temperature instability, respiratory problems, and changes in feeding habits or behavior. (See "Critical to Remember: Signs of Sepsis in the Newborn.") Early identification is important because shock can develop quickly.
12. Culture of specimens from blood, urine, skin lesions, and cerebral spinal fluid (identifies invading organism); complete blood count (identifies typical changes—decreased neutrophils, increased immature neutrophils [bands], and decreased platelets); immunoglobulin M (IgM) levels (identifies infection acquired in utero); C-reactive protein (shows an inflammatory process); chest radiography (rules out respiratory distress syndrome); blood glucose levels (unstable—high or low)
13. Blood is analyzed at the highest (peak) and lowest (trough) levels to provide a basis for any needed changes in dosage and to prevent toxic effects on body tissues.
14. If the diabetic woman has vascular changes, placental blood flow may be reduced, interfering with fetal growth. If the diabetic woman does not have vascular changes, she transfers large amounts of nutrients to the fetus. The fetus secretes large amounts of insulin to metabolize glucose, resulting in macrosomia.
15. (a) High fetal insulin levels interfere with surfactant production. (b) Maternal glucose supply ends at birth, but the infant temporarily continues a high level of insulin production. (c) Parathyroid hormone production is reduced. (d) Chronic fetal hypoxia stimulates production of more erythrocytes.
16. Length and head circumference are usually normal for the gestational age. The face is round, the skin is red, the body is obese, and muscle tone is poor. The infant is irritable and may have tremors when disturbed.
17. Signs include jitteriness, tremors, diaphoresis, tachypnea, low temperature, poor muscle tone, and low glucose screening test levels.
18. When excessive erythrocytes break down, bilirubin is released more quickly than it can be eliminated by the liver.
19. Infants appear hungry, but suck and swallow are poorly coordinated; hyperactive, increased muscle tone; regurgitation, vomiting, and diarrhea; signs typical of hypoglycemia but with a normal blood glucose level; restlessness; and irritability, failure to gain weight, and seizures.
20. Decreased environmental stimulation; avoid disturbing unnecessarily; swaddling; frequent feedings; protection of the skin
21. The infant has poor coordination of suck and swallow, reducing actual milk intake. At the same time, energy expenditure is high because of excess activity. Rapid respirations increase risk of aspiration if the infant is bottle-fed.
22. Decrease agitation by having feedings ready when the infant awakens. Swaddle the infant before beginning to feed. Feed in an area where distractions are limited and do not stimulate by talking or rocking during feedings. Support chin and cheeks to aid sucking, burp frequently.

23. Refer to text, pp. 826-828, to complete this exercise.
24. Blood flow to the lungs is decreased, and unoxygenated blood is mixed with oxygenated blood in the systemic circulation.

Check Yourself

1, c; 2, a; 3, d; 4, a; 5, b; 6, b; 7, a; 8, c; 9, a; 10, d

Case Study

1. The positive Coombs' test performed on cord blood obtained at birth indicates that antibodies from the mother have attached to the infant's red blood cells. Jaundice in the first 24 hours of life is pathological.
2. Monitoring of Steven's bilirubin level and skin color for increasing jaundice are essential related assessments.
3. The physician will probably order phototherapy at this time. The light causes bilirubin in the skin to change into a water-soluble form that can be excreted.
4. Nursing interventions related to phototherapy include the following:

- Cover the infant's closed eyes with patches to prevent damage if he is under phototherapy lights. Check placement of the patches hourly.
- Change the infant's position every 2 hours to distribute light exposure evenly over the skin surface. If a fiber-optic blanket is used, check its placement at the same intervals to ensure maximum exposure of the skin surface.
- Check the infant's temperature every 2 to 4 hours. Place a skin probe on the infant if he is in an incubator.
- Remove the infant from the lights only as necessary, such as for feeding or other care. This will not be necessary if a phototherapy blanket is used.
- Feed the infant every 2 to 3 hours to stimulate stool passage for excretion of bilirubin.
- Check the level of irradiance per agency policy to ensure optimum functioning.
- Use a reflectance photometer to measure transcutaneous bilirubin levels according to agency policy.

5. Side effects may include frequent loose, green stools; a tanned appearance in dark-skinned infants; skin rash; and temporary lactose intolerance.

Family Planning

Learning Activities

1. Why is the typical, or actual, failure rate of a contraceptive more useful than the theoretical failure rate?

2. How would you explain a failure rate of 15% for a contraceptive method? How can a woman decide whether that is good enough?

3. Why should a woman who is monogamous consider a contraceptive that provides protection from sexually transmitted diseases (STDs)?

4. Why should perimenopausal women use contraception and what kind of contraception is safe for them?

5. Why should a man have his semen analyzed after vasectomy?

6. How do estrogen-progestin oral contraceptives prevent conception?

7. How do progestin-only oral contraceptives prevent conception?

8. What teaching is appropriate in each area related to oral contraceptive use?
   a. Backup contraception

   b. Time of day

   c. Missed dose

   d. Possible pregnancy

   e. Use during lactation

   f. Other medications

9. What annual examinations should the woman have if she takes oral contraceptives?

10. Explain how to use the contraceptive patch and the vaginal ring.

11. List types of emergency contraception.

12. What teaching is important related to intrauterine device (IUD) use?

13. What are the two main advantages of barrier methods of contraception?

14. Why is the use of spermicide with condoms advisable?

15. What should the woman who uses spermicides be taught about douching?

16. Why is it essential to help the man or woman understand the difference between natural membrane condoms and latex condoms?

17. What is the major problem associated with the female condom?

18. At what times should the woman who uses a diaphragm for contraception have the fit checked?

19. What is the major problem in using natural family planning methods?

20. Complete the following table to describe advantages and disadvantages of each contraceptive method.

Method	Advantages	Disadvantages
Sterilization		
Hormone implant		
Hormone injection		
Oral contraception		
Emergency contraception		

Method	Advantages	Disadvantages
Transdermal patch		
Vaginal ring		
Intrauterine device		
Chemical barriers		
Male condom		
Female condom		
Sponge		

Method	Advantages	Disadvantages
Diaphragm		
Cervical cap		
Lea's shield		
Natural family planning		
Abstinence		
Breastfeeding		
Coitus interruptus		

Check Yourself

1. A woman is considering having a tubal ligation after she gives birth to her second child. The nurse should counsel her that
   a. She should wait until several months after birth to be certain the infant is healthy.
   b. The procedure should be considered permanent and irreversible.
   c. Sterilization is easier to perform 1 month after the postpartum period.
   d. She must sign informed consent by the sixth month of pregnancy.

2. Post-procedure teaching for a man who has had a vasectomy should include discussion that
   a. The first one or two urinations may be difficult after the procedure.
   b. A catheterized urine specimen should be obtained in 1 week.
   c. Levels of testosterone may fluctuate for the first few months.
   d. Contraception should be used until the semen is free of sperm.

3. What should the nurse know about hormone injection?
   a. Medroxyprogesterone (Depo-Provera) should be given intramuscularly.
   b. The injection site should be massaged vigorously.
   c. Injections should be given every 16 weeks.
   d. Amenorrhea usually occurs after the first month.

4. A woman decides to change from the diaphragm to Depo-Provera. Her last menstrual period ended 1 week ago. She should be taught that she should
   a. Take an oral contraceptive during this cycle only.
   b. Return in 1 week to have the hormone injection.
   c. Use another form of contraception for the first week.
   d. Expect more regular periods than when using the diaphragm.

5. How should a woman take oral contraceptives?
   a. On an empty stomach, with a full glass of water
   b. At approximately the same time each day
   c. Before every episode of intercourse
   d. In the morning and at bedtime

6. Choose the safety teaching related to oral contraceptives.
   a. Condoms should also be used if there is a chance of contracting an STD.
   b. Nausea and vomiting suggests that stroke may be imminent.
   c. Toxic shock syndrome is more likely when the pill is used.
   d. Increase fluids if urinary frequency or urgency occurs.

7. Teaching for a woman using the contraceptive sponge includes telling the woman that the sponge
   a. Must be replaced for repeated intercourse
   b. Can be left in place for up to 48 hours
   c. Should be wet with water before it is used
   d. Should remain in place for at least 4 hours

8. If the IUD strings are longer than usual, the woman should
   a. Know that this is expected when the IUD is first inserted
   b. Immediately have a Pap smear to rule out cervical cancer
   c. Take her temperature twice a day for 1 week
   d. See her physician and use another method of contraception

9. The major advantage of using a condom for contraception is that it
   a. Does not require monthly injections
   b. Reduces transmission of infections
   c. Can be placed several hours before intercourse
   d. May be incorporated as part of foreplay

10. In the symptothermal method of natural family planning
    a. Intercourse is avoided during the last half of the menstrual cycle.
    b. Weight gain, mittelschmerz, mucus, and bloating are assessed.
    c. Intercourse is unsafe if cervical mucus is thick and sticky.
    d. Temperature is taken orally every morning and evening.

Developing Insight

1. Have you known of adolescents who had erroneous beliefs such as those discussed on p. 840? Did you have any of these beliefs when you were an adolescent? How might you use age-appropriate counseling to correct this misinformation? How would you address the issue of confidentiality?

2. Practice how you might tactfully introduce the subject of contraception to an adolescent, a postpartum woman, and a woman in her mid 40s.

3. You are asked for contraceptive information by a 16-year-old girl, a 28-year-old woman with three children, and a 45-year-old woman with one child. If you could ask only two questions of each woman to help you find the best method for her, what questions would be most important? If you had to choose only two types of contraception to offer each, what would they be?

4. If you could design the perfect contraceptive method, what qualities would it have? Who would use it? How would it be obtained?

5. Oral contraceptives are available without prescription in many countries and may be available over the counter in the United States in the future. What are the advantages and disadvantages of this?

ANSWERS TO SELECTED QUESTIONS

Learning Activities

1. The typical failure rate reflects the way real people use a contraceptive and includes mistakes or inconsistencies of use. The theoretical failure rate refers to pregnancies that occur when the method is used perfectly every time it is used.
2. A failure rate of 15% means that 15 of every 100 women using the method are at risk for unintended pregnancy within a year. Whether this provides enough protection for the woman depends on how important she believes it is for her to avoid pregnancy.
3. Although the woman is monogamous, her partner may not be at this time or in the future. Either one of them might have an STD from a previous partner that is still infectious.
4. Perimenopausal women may ovulate even if they have indications of menopause. Healthy women in their 40s, who do not smoke, are not obese, or have no complications precluding use may take oral contraceptives. Women older than 35 years who smoke heavily or those older than 40 years who smoke at all should not use estrogen-containing contraceptives. They may use barrier or progestin-only contraceptives or sterilization safely.
5. Sperm may still be in the semen, and the man may be able to impregnate a woman for 3 months or more. Sperm specimens must show no sperm present to consider the man sterile.
6. They make the cervical mucus too thick for sperm to penetrate and suppress secretion of luteinizing and follicle-stimulating hormones, thereby preventing ovulation.
7. They thicken cervical mucus to prevent sperm penetration and make the endometrium unfavorable for implantation.
8. (a) Have a backup method readily available if doses are missed or if the woman decides to discontinue the method. Use a backup method for a week if the first month of pills are begun later than the first day of menses. (b) Take at the same time of day to maintain constant blood levels, maximize effectiveness, and reduce breakthrough bleeding. (c) See "Women Want to Know What to Do if an Oral Contraceptive Dose Is Missed". (d) Stop pills and get a sensitive pregnancy test; use a backup method. (e) Combination pills reduce milk production, and small amounts are transferred to milk; another contraceptive method is preferable; progestin-only contraception may be started 6 weeks after birth if breastfeeding exclusively or 3 weeks after birth if also using formula. (f) Interactions may alter the effectiveness of each medication; inform health care provider of all medications.
9. A blood pressure check yearly is essential when taking oral contraceptives. A Pap smear and breast examination is often recommended as part of a yearly checkup. Evaluate for side effects or adverse reactions at the time of any examination.
10. The patch should be applied to clean, dry, healthy skin and worn continuously for a week, when it is replaced with a new patch placed at a different site. After 3 weeks, the woman omits the patch for 1 week. The vaginal ring is inserted into the vagina and left in place for 3 weeks and then removed for 1 week. During the patch- or ring-free week, menses will occur.
11. The usual method is to take 2 tablets that have a high dose of progestin (Plan B) within 120 hours of unprotected intercourse. High doses of combined oral contraceptives may also be taken. Insertion of the copper T 380A IUD within 5 days is another option.
12. Check for the string monthly after the menstrual period and if there is cramping or unexpected bleeding, which may indicate expulsion. See health care provider if strings are longer or shorter than before. Report signs of infection or pregnancy. Return yearly for a Pap smear and check for anemia.
13. Avoidance of systemic hormones and some protection from STDs
14. The spermicide increases protection by adding a chemical barrier to the mechanical barrier of the condom and lubricates the condom to reduce tearing.
15. Avoid douching for at least 6 hours after intercourse to avoid washing the protection away.
16. Natural membrane condoms allow passage of viruses and do not provide protection from STDs. Latex condoms provide better protection against STDs.
17. It is less effective (typical failure rate of 21%).
18. She should have it checked yearly, after a weight gain or loss of more than 20%, or after a pregnancy.
19. Any error in predicting ovulation or safe times for intercourse can result in pregnancy.
20. Complete this table as you read the text in this chapter.

Check Yourself

1, b; 2, d; 3, a; 4, c; 5, b; 6, a; 7, c; 8, d; 9, b; 10, b

CHAPTER 32 | Infertility

Learning Activities

1. Match each term with its definition (a-h).

_____ Diethylstilbestrol

_____ Hypospadias

_____ Hysterosalpingogram

_____ Myoma

_____ Postcoital test

_____ Pregnancy wastage

_____ Sperm swim-up

_____ Transcervical balloon tuboplasty

a. Repeated loss of pregnancy before the fetus is mature enough to survive

b. Procedure to unblock fallopian tubes without using a surgical incision

c. Urethral opening on the underside of the penis

d. Hormone that has been associated with cervical or uterine abnormalities

e. Benign muscle tumor

f. Imaging studies to evaluate the structure and patency of the uterus and fallopian tubes

g. Evaluation of cervical mucus and sperm function after intercourse at the time of ovulation

h. Procedure to capture the sperm most likely to achieve fertilization in a therapeutic insemination

2. List factors that can impair the ability of sperm to fertilize the ovum.

3. List factors that can impair normal erections.

4. List causes of abnormal ejaculation.

5. List factors that can impair the function of seminal fluid.

6. List factors that can disrupt the woman's hormonal secretions that are needed to achieve pregnancy.

7. List factors that can impair normal ovulation.

8. List factors that can impair structure and function of the fallopian tubes.

9. List factors that can obstruct or impair function in the woman's cervix.

10. List factors that may be associated with repeated pregnancy loss.

11. Describe nursing care associated with each of the more common diagnostic tests for infertility. Include male and female evaluations as appropriate for some tests.
   a. Ovulation prediction, including basal body temperature

   b. Hormone evaluations (give examples)

   c. Ultrasound

   d. Hysterosalpingogram

   e. Endometrial biopsy

   f. Semen analysis

   g. Testicular biopsy

   h. Sperm penetration assay

   i. Postcoital testing

12. Describe two complications associated with medications given to induce ovulation.
   a.

   b.

13. What are some reasons that therapeutic insemination may be chosen?

14. What precautions lessen the risk that a man will transmit infection or genetic disorders when he donates his sperm?

15. Complete the following table comparing in vitro fertilization (IVF), gamete intrafallopian transfer (GIFT), zygote intrafallopian transfer (ZIFT), and intracytoplasmic sperm injection (ICSI). Have you or anyone you know had any of these assisted reproductive techniques done to improve chances of conception?

Procedure	Description	Advantages	Disadvantages
IVF			
GIFT			
ZIFT			
ICSI			

Check Yourself

1. When teaching a woman fertility awareness, the nurse should emphasize that the basal body temperature
   a. Is the average temperature taken each morning
   b. Should be recorded each morning before any activity
   c. Has the highest degree of accuracy in predicting ovulation
   d. Can be taken with any digital thermometer

2. At ovulation, the basal body temperature usually
   a. Rises abruptly and then falls 1 or 2 days after menstruation starts
   b. Falls and remains low for the last half of the cycle
   c. Is higher during the first half of the cycle than in the last half
   d. Falls just before ovulation and is higher during the last half

3. Cervical mucus at ovulation should be
   a. Thin and slippery and should stretch to at least 6 cm
   b. Cloudy with a mild odor and should stretch to at least 6 cm
   c. Thick, clear, and of a large quantity
   d. Thin and tinged with a small amount of blood

4. Choose the correct instructions for a man who must provide a semen sample.
   a. After collecting the sample in a condom, refrigerate it until it is transported to the laboratory.
   b. Masturbation is the only way a good sample can be obtained.
   c. Keep the sample near the body, and transport it to the laboratory within 1 hour.
   d. Do not take any regularly scheduled drugs for 3 days before obtaining the sample.

5. A woman who is taking clomiphene citrate (Clomid) phones the infertility clinic and says that she has some nausea each morning and frequency of urination. She suspects that she may be pregnant. The correct nursing response is to
   a. Tell her that pregnancy cannot be determined until she misses her next period
   b. Have her come to the clinic promptly for sensitive pregnancy testing
   c. Explain that she should have a pregnancy test after she completes this drug cycle
   d. Reassure her that her symptoms are commonly seen in women who take this drug

Developing Insight

1. What is your opinion about monetary compensation for a woman who is a surrogate mother and contributes her ovum to the child? What if she is a gestational surrogate and carries the fetus to term but does not contribute a gamete to him or her?

2. Should compensation be different for male sperm donors and females who donate their ovum and carry the fetus? Why?

3. What are your feelings about blastomere analysis to identify genetic defects before implantation of an embryo that results from an assisted reproductive technology procedure? Should an embryo that has an identified defect be implanted? If it is to be discarded, what is your moral and ethical view on the situation?

4. Should health insurance cover all infertility diagnostic studies and therapy? If not, which ones should not be covered? Does your own health insurance provide infertility coverage?

5. Should public assistance funds such as Medicaid cover infertility therapy? Why or why not? What if the woman seeking infertility therapy now has more children than she can support, with or without a partner?

ANSWERS TO SELECTED QUESTIONS

Learning Activities

1. d, c, f, e, g, a, h, b
2. Abnormal hormone stimulation; acute or chronic illness; infections of the genital tract; anatomic abnormalities; exposure to toxins; therapeutic treatments for cancer or other illness; excessive alcohol intake; drug ingestion; elevated scrotal temperature; antibodies produced by the man or the woman that alter structure, function, or motion of sperm
3. Disorders of the central or autonomic nervous system, spinal cord disorders, peripheral vascular disease, drugs
4. Diabetes, neurologic disorders, surgery that affects sympathetic nerve function, drugs (therapeutic or illicit), some spinal cord injuries, anatomic abnormalities, excessive alcohol intake, psychological factors
5. Obstruction, inflammation, or infection in the genital tract
6. Cranial tumors, stress, obesity, anorexia, systemic disease, ovarian or endocrine abnormalities, advancing age
7. Cancer chemotherapy, excessive alcohol intake, cigarette smoking
8. Infections, endometriosis or surgery that causes adhesions, congenital anomalies
9. Polyps or cervical damage from surgical procedures, hormonal imbalances, cervical damage secondary to infection or other factors
10. Chromosome abnormalities, cervical or uterine abnormalities, hormone imbalances that disrupt implantation and establishment of the placenta, diabetes, immunologic rejection of the embryo, lupus erythematosus, environmental toxins, infections
11. Refer to text, pp. 868-869, including Table 32-1 (p. 863) and Procedure 31-1 (pp. 855-856), to complete this exercise.
12. (a) The risk for multifetal pregnancies increases because multiple ova may be released and thus fertilized. (b) Ovarian hyperstimulation syndrome can cause exudation of fluid into the woman's peritoneal and pleural cavities.
13. Low sperm count, genetic defect carried by the male, woman's desire for a biologic child without having a male partner, avoiding cervical and immunologic incompatibilities
14. A personal and family health history is taken; questions are asked about social habits and personality. Other tests include a physical examination and laboratory studies, including those for common genetic defects. Donor sperm is frozen and held for 6 months before use, and the donor is retested for human immunodeficiency virus (HIV) during this time.
15. Refer to text, pp. 871-873, to complete this question.

Check Yourself

1, b (refer to Procedure 31-1, pp. 855-856); 2, d; 3, a; 4, c; 5, b

Learning Activities

1. Match each term with its definition (a-d).

_____ body mass index (BMI)   a. Analysis of cervical tissue for disease

_____ BSE   b. Calculation to determine whether a person is of healthy weight

_____ FOBT   c. Monthly breast examination by a woman

_____ Pap test   d. Test to identify possible colorectal cancer

2. What is the purpose of the Women's Health Initiative?

3. Why should a women's health nurse specifically ask a woman about her use of complementary or alternative therapies, such as botanical preparations, when conducting a health screening?

4. Define overweight and obesity. What problems are associated with these conditions?

5. When should breast self-examination (BSE) be performed?

6. What are the current recommendations for screening mammography (American Cancer Society and American College of Obstetricians and Gynecologists)?

7. What is the recommendation for vulvar self-examination?

8. What preparation should a woman make for a pelvic examination with a Pap test?

9. Who is offered the fecal occult blood testing (FOBT)? What are the preparations for the test, and how are samples obtained?

10. How often should a colonoscopy be performed? Why may it be performed more frequently?

Check Yourself

1. Breast self-examination should be performed using the
   a. Palm of the left hand to palpate the right breast in a wedge pattern
   b. Horizontal pattern to palpate across both breasts at one pass
   c. Middle three fingertips of the left hand to palpate the right breast
   d. Thumb of the opposite hand to palpate each breast in a circular pattern

2. The nurse practitioner is seeing a 58-year-old woman for her yearly well-woman examination (WWE). The woman complains that, "I'm getting wider with age I guess, but I haven't gained any weight. I just have more trouble buttoning my pants and skirts now." The nurse-practitioner should initially
   a. Encourage the woman to develop an exercise plan that will work for her.
   b. Determine whether the woman's height has changed since the previous year.
   c. Ask the woman whether she has any persistent gastrointestinal or chest discomfort.
   d. Calculate the woman's BMI and compare with her previous visit.

3. A woman will have screening for fecal occult blood. Choose the correct instructions.
   a. Do not take nonsteroidal antiinflammatory drugs (NSAIDs) for 1 week before collecting the samples.
   b. Eat two servings of red meat each day for 3 days before obtaining the samples.
   c. Collect a small sample of stool from the first stool expelled each morning for 3 days.
   d. Refrigerate the samples until they can be returned to the laboratory for testing.

4. A 25-year-old woman is being seen for her first WWE at the clinic. Her vital signs are normal, height is 64 inches, and weight is 160 lb. Select the most important area of focus with her initial interview that is indicated by this basic information.
   a. Number of pregnancies and their outcome; mode of delivery
   b. Type and quantity of food eaten on an average day
   c. Personal history of sexually transmitted diseases and number of partners
   d. Family history of weight problems, diabetes, or heart disease

5. A 45-year-old woman is having a WWE. Her last menstrual period was 2 years ago. In addition to the Pap test, the nurse-practitioner plans to draw blood for a complete blood count (CBC), a complete metabolic profile (CMP), and a lipid profile. The woman asks why the lipid profile has been added to her usual annual laboratory tests. The best reply of the nurse practitioner is that
   a. The risk for coronary artery disease is higher after menopause and measures to reduce the risk may be needed.
   b. Excess weight after menopause may occur if the lipids are not well balanced, and diet changes may be indicated.
   c. High triglyceride levels reduce her risk for osteoporosis and she can delay the bone density tests another year.
   d. Women often have a high cholesterol level after menopause that increases their risk for breast cancer.

Developing Insight

1. Do you think that yearly WWEs are cost-effective in light of the high cost of health care in the United States? Is it reasonable to cover the annual WWE at 100% under public or private health plans? Explain the rationale for your answers.

2. You are giving influenza vaccine in a public clinic. One woman brings her older mother but refuses an injection for herself. When asked the reason she replies that "I had a flu shot last year and caught it a few days later anyway. It didn't do me any good." What teaching is reasonable for this woman?

3. Calculate the BMI for each adult height and weight listed here. A calculator is available at <u>www.cdc.gov</u> for adults and children or teens or you may find one in most nutrition or other nursing textbooks.

a. 5 feet, 5 inches; 215 lb

b. 6 feet, 2 inches; 200 lb

c. 5 feet, 10 inches; 135 lb

ANSWERS TO SELECTED QUESTIONS

Learning Activities

1. b, c, d, a

2. The Women's Health Initiative will continue long-term studies of the top causes of death and disability in older women of every race (cardiovascular disease, breast cancer, colorectal cancer, osteoporosis) to 2010.

3. People who use complementary or alternative therapies often do not consider these to be drugs, although many have active ingredients. They may not mention the fact that they use the therapies even though some may interfere with medically prescribed therapy.

4. Overweight, BMI 25 to 25.9; obesity, BMI 30 to 30.9. Problems associated with overweight and obesity: diabetes, hypertension, coronary artery disease.

5. Monthly by all women older than 20 years; 1 week after the menstrual period begins or on a specific day of the month if the woman is not menstruating

6. American Cancer Society: yearly for women 40 years and older. American College of Obstetricians and Gynecologists: every 1 to 2 years for women age 40 to 49 years; yearly after 50 years. Earlier or more frequent screenings may be recommended for women at high risk for breast cancer.

7. Monthly for women older than age 18 years and by those younger than age 18 years if sexually active

8. Schedule the examination between menstrual periods. Do not douche or have sexual intercourse for at least 48 hours before the examination. Do not use vaginal medications, sprays, or deodorants.

9. FOBT is a yearly screening for colorectal cancer beginning at age 50 years. Preparation for the test includes avoidance of vitamin C, aspirin, nonsteroidal antiinflammatory drugs (NSAIDs), red meat, raw fruits and vegetables, and horseradish. A specimen should be collected from three consecutive stools, and the slides should be returned within 4 to 6 days as directed.

10. Colonoscopy may be recommended yearly for those with a family history of colon cancer, but otherwise every 10 years after age 50.

Check Yourself

1, c; 2, b; 3, a; 4, d; 5, a

Developing Insight

3. a. 35.8 BMI, obese; b. 25.7 BMI, overweight; c. 19.4 BMI, normal

Women's Health Problems

Learning Activities

1. Match each term with its definition (a-g).

_____ Estrogen receptor-positive cancer   a. Thickening of normal tissue

_____ Fibrosis   b. Abnormal proliferation of normal cells

_____ Hyperplasia   c. Small elevation or protuberance in tissue

_____ Induced abortion   d. Swelling caused by obstruction of lymphatic vessels or nodes

_____ Lymphedema   e. Often called "cramps"

_____ Papilloma   f. Voluntary interruption of a pregnancy

_____ Primary dysmenorrhea   g. Malignant tissue that is stimulated by estrogen

2. Describe the signs, symptoms, and treatment for each benign breast disorder.
   a. Fibrocystic breast changes

   b. Fibroadenoma

   c. Ductal ectasia

   d. Intraductal papilloma

3. Describe major management methods for breast cancer.

4. List symptoms of a myocardial infarction (MI) that a woman is likely to have that may differ from the classic MI symptoms.

5. List the major risk factors for coronary artery disease (CAD) in women.

6. What are the current nutrition recommendations related to cardiovascular health?

7. What are current activity recommendations to maintain heart health?

8. Define each type of amenorrhea, and give common causes for each.
   a. Primary

   b. Secondary

9. List common causes of abnormal uterine bleeding.

10. What is the nurse's role in caring for women who have abnormal uterine bleeding?

11. What treatment is typical for each type of cyclic pelvic pain?
   a. Mittelschmerz

   b. Primary dysmenorrhea

   c. Endometriosis

12. What nursing measures are appropriate when a woman has premenstrual syndrome (PMS)?

13. Explain the purpose for each technique that may be used in medical termination of pregnancy, and state any side or adverse effects, if applicable.

Procedure	Purpose	Side or Adverse Effects
Vacuum aspiration		
Dilation and removal of fetus/placenta		
Laminaria	Not applicable	
Prostaglandin E$_2$		
Oxytocin		

14. Describe how each drug can cause abortion and at what time during pregnancy, if applicable.
    a. Mifepristone (Mifeprex, RU 486)

    b. Methotrexate (Folex, Mexate)

    c. Misoprostol (Cytotec)

15. Why should a woman promptly report unexpected uterine bleeding after menopause?

16. What is the purpose of giving estrogen with progestin to relieve the symptoms of menopause?

17. Describe benefits and risks that effect hormone replacement therapy at menopause. Include both estrogen-only replacement and estrogen-progesterone replacement. Identify reasons that the hormone therapy should be prescribed with caution or is contraindicated.

Type of Hormone	Benefits of Therapy	Risks of Therapy	Replacement Therapy
Estrogen-only replacement			
Estrogen-progesterone replacement			

18. What alternative therapies exist, including botanical preparations, for the woman who does not want to take estrogen or for whom it is contraindicated?

19. What signs occur when a woman has osteoporosis? What are the most common fracture sites?

20. Describe drug therapy for osteoporosis.

21. How should a woman be taught to perform the Kegel exercise? How frequently should she do it?

22. What screening tests may be used to identify female reproductive tract cancers early?

23. Complete the following table on sexually transmitted diseases as you read your text.

Disease	Signs and Symptoms	Treatment	Teaching
Candidiasis			
Trichomoniasis			
Bacterial vaginosis			
Chlamydia			
Gonorrhea			
Syphilis			
Herpes genitalis			
Condylomata acuminata			
Acquired immuno-deficiency syndrome			

24. How does pelvic inflammatory disease occur? What are its results?

Check Yourself

1. Your friend calls to tell you that she noticed a small amount of nipple retraction in her right nipple when she was showering. As a nurse, you should advise her to
   a. Perform a complete breast self-examination to determine whether any lumps are present
   b. Wait until 1 week after her next menstrual period and then do a breast self-examination
   c. Note if there is any change in the amount of nipple retraction for 2 weeks
   d. See her primary health care provider for a professional examination

2. Preoperative nursing care for the woman anticipating a modified radical mastectomy for breast cancer includes teaching about
   a. Restricted arm movement on the operative side for 2 weeks after surgery
   b. Drainage tubes that will remove fluid that accumulates under the operative area
   c. A small dressing applied to the operative site
   d. A hospital stay of 3 to 4 days

3. To relieve her menstrual cramps, a woman should be taught to take ibuprofen
   a. Within 8 hours of the onset of menstruation
   b. During the week before the expected onset of her period
   c. Around the clock for 2 to 3 days at the onset of menstruation
   d. On an empty stomach before the pain becomes severe

4. Your friend is having hot flashes as she enters menopause. She is interested in hormone replacement to improve these symptoms but is fearful of breast cancer. As a nurse, you should tell her that
   a. Her physician or nurse practitioner can evaluate her risk and help her make a better decision.
   b. The risk of breast cancer is very small for women who are younger than the age of 60 years when menstrual periods stop.
   c. Taking the estrogen with progestin will reduce the risk for estrogen-induced breast cancer.
   d. The benefits of estrogen replacement therapy far outweigh any risks associated with it.

5. When teaching a woman to take alendronate (Fosamax), the nurse should tell her to
   a. Take the tablet with a full glass of milk to prevent gastric pain.
   b. Take the medication at night just before bedtime to promote absorption.
   c. Reduce intake of calcium supplements after being on the drug for 1 month.
   d. Remain upright for at least 30 minutes after taking the drug each morning.

6. If a woman is taking aspirin, 81 mg daily, after a myocardial infarction, the nurse should be observant for problems related to
   a. Calcium loss and fractures
   b. Urinary tract infection
   c. Premature loss of memory function
   d. Bruising and evidence of bleeding disorders

7. To reduce the risk for toxic shock syndrome, women should be taught to
   a. Avoid changing tampons until they are thoroughly saturated
   b. Use a diaphragm with spermicidal jelly during the menstrual period
   c. Wash hands thoroughly before inserting a tampon or diaphragm into the vagina
   d. Limit the use of superabsorbent tampons to the times when flow is heavy

Developing Insight

1. Talk with a woman who has had breast cancer about her feelings on learning the diagnosis and during the wait between diagnosis and treatment.

2. When caring for people who have experienced age-related fractures, such as a hip fracture, note how many of them are older and female. Do you note any other adverse effects of osteoporosis other than fractures?

3. Look around you at the number of women who apparently have lost height or have other effects of osteoporosis. Describe what you see in the women to make you think that osteoporosis may be to blame.

4. Do you see risk behaviors for osteoporosis in young women? What are they?

ANSWERS TO SELECTED QUESTIONS

Learning Activities

1. g, a, b, f, d, c, e
2. (a) Thickening or multiple smooth, well-delineated nodules; tenderness and pain noticeable during the latter half of the menstrual cycle but less during pregnancy; aspiration of clear fluid normal and often not repeated; definitive studies such as mammogram and ultrasound imaging, fine-needle aspiration (FNA), or surgical biopsy rule out malignancy; avoiding caffeine and other stimulants and limiting salt intake may help. (b) Firm, hard, freely movable nodules that may or may not be tender and do not change during the menstrual cycle; observation with possible biopsy or excision followed by pathologic analysis. (c) Firm, irregular mass with enlarged axillary nodes and nipple retraction and discharge; surgical biopsy; no treatment if ductal ectasia is confirmed. (d) Serous or serosanguineous discharge from the nipple; excision of mass and duct with analysis of discharge to rule out malignancy.
3. Surgical therapy removes part or all of the breast plus lymph node analysis to determine cancer's spread. Adjuvant therapy may include radiation and chemotherapy, including hormonal therapy and immunotherapy. Breast reconstruction assists in the psychological recovery.
4. Fatigue; weakness; angina or pain at rest; dyspnea, sometimes paroxysmal nocturnal dyspnea; dizziness, faintness, lightheadedness; upper abdominal pain, heartburn, loss of appetite; nausea, vomiting, sweating; pain in the upper body other than the chest (arm, neck, back, jaw, throat, teeth)
5. Cigarette smoking, hypertension, dyslipidemia, diabetes, excessive body weight, sedentary lifestyle, poor nutrition, postmenopausal, family history
6. Fat should make up a maximum of 30% of daily calories and saturated fat a maximum of 10% of daily calories; cholesterol less than 200 mg/day. Fish (especially fatty fish), 2 servings/week; high fruit and vegetable intake, low-fat dairy products, and limiting salt and alcohol intake are recommended on a daily basis.
7. At least 30 minutes of moderate daily physical exercise can control weight, control blood pressure, and improve the lipid profile and glucose levels.
8. (a) Absence of first menses within 2 years of breast development, usually between ages 10 and 16 years. Causes: Turner's syndrome (single X chromosome); chemotherapy or radiation therapy; low body weight; chronic stress; hypothyroidism; central nervous system diseases; drug use; anatomic abnormalities of the uterus, vagina, or hymen; congenital enzyme abnormalities. (b) Cessation of menses for at least 6 months in a woman who has established menstruation. Causes: pregnancy; systemic diseases such as diabetes, tuberculosis; hormonal imbalances; low weight; stress; systemic illness; poor nutrition; oral contraceptives; antidepressants; tumors of the ovary, pituitary, or adrenal gland.
9. Pregnancy complications; anatomic lesions (benign or malignant); drug-induced bleeding ("breakthrough bleeding"); systemic disorders such as diabetes; uterine myomas; hypothyroidism; failure to ovulate
10. Urge the woman to seek medical help. Help the woman record bleeding episodes and associated symptoms. Teach about needed lifestyle changes, such as adequate diet and stress reduction. Provide information about diagnostic procedures that may be recommended.
11. (a) Mild analgesics and reassurance about the cause of the discomfort. (b) Oral contraceptives and prostaglandin-inhibiting drugs such as nonsteroidal antiinflammatory drugs (NSAIDs); rest or application of warmth. (c) Oral contraceptives, medroxyprogesterone, danazol, or a gonadotropin-releasing hormone agonist to suppress endometrial tissue growth; hysterectomy with bilateral salpingo-oophorectomy; lysis of adhesions and laser vaporization of the lesions.
12. Urge the woman to seek a thorough examination to diagnose her problem properly. Teach dietary changes, exercises, stress management, and techniques to promote sleep and rest (refer to "Women Want to Know: How to Relieve Symptoms of PMS," p. 909, to complete the exercise).
13. Refer to text, pp. 909-911, to complete this exercise.
14. (a) Inhibits progesterone; can be used through the ninth week of gestation. (b) Interferes with DNA synthesis. (c) Causes uterine contractions; can be used up to second trimester; may be used in conjunction with other medications used to medically terminate pregnancy.
15. Postmenopausal bleeding suggests endometrial cancer.
16. Estrogen alone would cause endometrial hyperplasia if the woman has her uterus.
17. Refer to text, pp. 912-914.
18. Phytoestrogens are contained in products made of soybeans, such as tofu, soy cheese, soy milk, and soy flour. Other botanical preparations include black cohosh, chasteberry, and dong quai (see text for precautions and interactions). Water-soluble lubricants, Kegel exercises, adequate water intake, and front-to-back cleansing or wiping of the vaginal area reduce infections and discomforts of the vagina and bladder.
19. Initially, no signs or symptoms are present. When they appear, they include loss of height, back pain, the "dowager's hump," disappearance of the waistline, and abdominal

protrusion. Fractures of the hip, vertebrae, and wrist are the most common osteoporosis-associated breaks.

20. Estrogen replacement to limit loss (based on evaluation of her risk level); calcium replacement with vitamin D; exercise (ideally muscle strengthening and high impact); medications such as calcitonin, alendronate, risedronate, raloxifene, and zoledronic acid.

21. She may be taught how to perform the Kegel exercise while urinating, but the nurse should emphasize that it is not ordinarily performed while urinating. She should be taught to exhale and keep the mouth open to avoid bearing down. She should contract the pelvic muscles as if stopping the flow of urine during urination. Each contraction should be held for at least 3 seconds, building to at least 10 seconds each. Variations in frequency exist but range from 24 to 45 times each day with a relaxation period of 10 seconds between each pelvic muscle contraction.

22. Periodic pelvic examinations, Pap tests, ultrasonography, and tests for tumor markers; diagnostic procedures such as endometrial biopsy and colposcopy

23. Refer to text, pp. 921-924, to complete this exercise.

24. Bacteria, often *Chlamydia trachomatis* and *Neisseria gonorrhoeae,* ascend through the cervix into the upper reproductive tract and pelvic cavity. Here the organisms cause a chronic inflammatory response that causes scarring of the fallopian tubes and adhesions near the tubes. Infertility is a common result.

Check Yourself

1. d; 2, b; 3, c; 4, a; 5, d; 6, d; 7, c